HAVE YOU WONDERED . . .

IS IT TIME FOR ME TO GET FERTILITY
TREATMENTS?

DOES AGE AFFECT A MAN TOO?

WILL MY INSURANCE COVER FERTILITY
TREATMENTS?

WHAT ARE THE CHANCES I'LL
CONCEIVE TWINS?

WHAT DO FERTILITY DRUGS DO TO MY BODY?

DO THEY INCREASE THE RISK OF CANCER?

ARE THERE NATURAL REMEDIES I CAN TRY?

AS LONG AS I GET MY PERIOD, AM I FERTILE?

CAN I GET PREGNANT IF I AM PAST
MENOPAUSE?

IF I HAD MY TUBES TIED, CAN IT BE REVERSED?

WHERE CAN I FIND A SPERM BANK?

GET THE ANSWERS IN . . .
101 ANSWERS TO YOUR FERTILITY QUESTIONS

101 ANSWERS TO YOUR FERTILITY QUESTIONS

Michelle Arnot

Foreword by
Dr. Lawrence Grunfeld, M.D., FACOG

A Dell Book

Published by
Dell Publishing
a division of
Bantam Doubleday Dell Publishing Group, Inc.
1540 Broadway
New York, New York 10036

Important Note: This book is not intended as a substitute
for the medical advice of a physician. The reader should
consult a physician with respect to any symptoms which
may require diagnosis or medical attention.

ISBN: 0-440-22383-0

Printed in the United States of America

Published simultaneously in Canada

November 1997

10   9   8   7   6   5   4   3   2   1

WCD

In memory of the artists
Ewald and Jackie-Yaffa Arnot,
my parents

ACKNOWLEDGMENTS

The author extends her sincere gratitude to the patients who inspired the focus of this book, as well as to the professional organizations and doctors who provided the research for the answers. Foremost among these are Resolve, The American Society for Reproductive Medicine, and the Center for Medical Consumers in New York City. For generously sharing their time and expertise, she is grateful to the eminent reproductive endocrinologists Dr. Larry Grunfeld, currently associated with the St. Barnabas program in New Jersey, and Dr. Isaac Kligman of the New York Hospital–Cornell Medical Center.

A personal note of thanks to Nancy Gallt at William Morrow for suggesting the format of the project and to Craig Virden at BDD for directing its course. For the introduction to the Internet, thank you to Web site designer Jacqueline Arnot. For serving as first reader, eternal gratitude to her husband, Roger Brown. Finally, the author thanks Mary Anne Erickson for setting the example, and the medical profession for developing the miraculous technology that is explained in the pages ahead.

CONTENTS

PART II: THE WORKUP

Questions About Your Fertility Checkup

Male Factors

Female Factors

PART III: CAUSES
**Questions About Underlying Reasons
for Infertility**

PART IV: TREATMENTS
Conventional Medical Methods

Unconventional Methods

PART V: CONCERNS

What is the current medical wisdom on the subject of . . .

PART VI: RESOURCES
Where to Find Medical Referrals

FOREWORD

by Lawrence Grunfeld, M.D., FACOG
associated with the Institute of Reproductive
Medicine and Science
at St. Barnabas Medical Center

By definition the choice to pursue parenthood through medical intervention is a strenuous undertaking. Educating yourself on this subject is the best antidote to stress, which is how reading this book can give you a leg up. Knowledge is power: The more you understand about the human reproductive process, the better you can manage your treatment. In buying this book, you have taken the first step in finding out what has been preventing conception. The good news is that research and development are on your side. Whereas even five years ago a biological family was not possible for many couples who visited my office, the latest technology has raised success rates for in vitro fertilization in our practice to 50% for women under the age of 40.

Contrary to popular belief, stress is not a cause of infertility, but infertility does cause stress. After a lifetime of good health a sudden shift to patienthood can be a bit jarring. The prospect of injecting potent prescription drugs or lying on an operating table may be more than you bargained for when you made the decision to start a family. Then there's the added burden of learning the language of treatment. IUI versus IVF, LH versus FSH tend to become one unappetizing alphabet soup at first. At a time when you need to be clearheaded in order to make decisions that will affect the rest of your life, protecting your equilibrium becomes a top priority.

By now you may have had the initial interview with your specialist. If so, then it shouldn't surprise you to learn that on average a patient absorbs just 20% of the information shared during that visit. Each aspect under discussion may set off a volley of distracting thoughts: the financing, the time commitment, the medications, the ensuing emotions. All this work to ensure the successful meeting of a single sperm with a single egg! What a complex business this rendezvous has become. It's a good idea to jot down notes during the consultation so that you have something to refer to later. Undoubtedly two heads recall more than one; both partners should be present at the initial interview since each will tune in differently.

The purpose of this book is to address the most commonly asked questions that fertility doctors answer each day and provide you with a base of knowledge that will serve you throughout your treatment. Using *101 Answers to Your Fertility Questions* as a resource will help you select knowledgeably from the menu of available medical options. The better your grasp of current scientific technology, the better equipped you will be to manage your treatment.

Diagnostic Testing

Each fertility program requires a set of standard workup tests. In our practice we begin by measuring the function of the essentials: semen, uterus and fallopian tubes, and ovaries. Once the medical team reviews the results of the man's semen analysis and the woman's blood test results and detects the function of the uterus and fallopian tubes, a determination is made on where the problem lies. On the basis of the index of initial indications, your doctor may be able to tailor your workup to suit any suspected underlying factor.

Until you have a definitive diagnosis, there's no need to stop trying to conceive on your own. First, you must focus on timing. Let go of the myth of precision. Coordinating intercourse to precede ovulation is the most important aspect of successful conception. A woman's most fertile day is just before the luteinizing hormone (LH) surge that occurs halfway into her cycle. If you're using an ovulation kit, that translates to the day the tab changes color. Intercourse every other day two to four days before the surge should ensure that one sperm has ample opportunity to fertilize the egg, provided that both gametes are healthy and that the fallopian tubes are open and receptive. Following the surge, pick up the pace by having intercourse daily for three days. Secondly, modify your intake of coffee and alcohol, and avoid exposure to such toxic materials as herbicides. These are known to have a negative impact on human fertility.

For every medical test that is recommended, ask your doctor if there are alternatives. Since tests are often expensive and possibly invasive, it pays in every sense to explore your options. Select carefully and consider your choices. As results come back, understand how they resonate in your case and devise a plan for how you will proceed for each possible outcome.

Treatment

Since the birth of the first so-called test-tube baby in 1978, in vitro technology has evolved quickly. In the nineties the field has truly exploded. Today's IVF technology compared with what it was in 1991 is like comparing a Ferrari with a bicycle. Major strides have been made every step of the way, from the way embryos are created to the formula of the medium in the petri dish to the design of the catheter used in embryo transfers. With the miracle of intracytoplasmic sperm injection (ICSI) the field of sperm micromanipulation has eliminated male factor infertility altogether. Right now we are on the brink of revolutionizing fertility drug treatments with the use of GnRH antagonists. This new class of drugs will give the reproductive endocrinologist complete control over the woman's ovulation, without the unpleasant side effects caused by current medications.

The couple in treatment needs to be up-to-date on the available procedures and where to find the best appropriate care. Since "corrective" surgery may have a negative impact on fertility, the qualifications of the surgeon are key when operations are indicated.

Besides a general understanding of medical techniques, the fertility patient needs to clarify basic expectations of what a specialist can do. First of all, you should know that doctors cannot turn back the clock. It's a mistake to believe that you can safely postpone childbearing beyond age 35. Today's fertility patients are considering starting families at an age when most of their mothers had completed this chapter of their lives. If you know you want a biological family, it's best not to delay. The image of motherhood may have changed since the 1950s, but the biology of conception hasn't.

Science now supports the notion that a woman's fertility is prime in her twenties, dropping off after age 30 with precipitous drops at 35 and 40. Of course donor eggs offer an excellent prognosis to the older patient who is receptive to taking this route.

Secondly, the patient must have a full understanding up front of what insurance will cover in treatment. Especially when the carrier has set a lifetime cap, you need to know your budget parameters so that you can spend wisely. While the specialist will work with you to contain costs, you cannot expect the practitioner to commit insurance fraud.

It's important to invest some time and energy in interviewing a fertility program before you enroll. As with any investment, you want the satisfaction of knowing that you made the best decision for you. Although you may be eager to get on with treatment, a bit of research can pay off in the long run. The place to begin your review is the laboratory. At this juncture the embryologists are driving the field forward. With the more experienced labs raising IVF success rates up as high as 50% for women under 40 in some clinics, the patient as consumer needs to investigate whether the lab offers the most up-to-date services.

As a practitioner in this young, exciting medical field, I derive great personal satisfaction in working with my colleagues in order to offer a couple the gift of a pregnancy. While certain issues have yet to be resolved (specifically reducing the occurrence of twins and triplets because of drug therapy), nearly 30,000 American children have been born to date thanks to fertility treatment. Despite this good news, new patients often confide the secret sense they have that infertility is a punishment for past behavior. This is absolutely not the case. Infertility is not a new development; it has been reported since biblical times. The difference is that it was once incurable and now, as we enter the twenty-first century, infertility has become a treatable condition. With this inspiration in mind, let this book guide you through treatment.

INTRODUCTION

FACT: About 5,000,000 couples are infertile in the United States today. Fertility technology will help only half this population.

FACT: Sexually transmitted disease (STD) is responsible for causing infertility for one in four couples of reproductive age in the United States.

FACT: Fertility drugs help only 10% of infertile couples with unexplained infertility.

FACT: In vitro fertility treatment costs between $10,000 and $20,000 per cycle.

FACT: After age 35 the quality of a woman's eggs begins to deteriorate significantly.

FACT: One in two eggs exhibits chromosomal abnormalities for women over 40.

FACT: Modern technology is not yet able to produce adequate pregnancy rates in a woman over 43 *with her own eggs*. She may get pregnant with a younger woman's eggs.

FACT: Assisted reproductive technology (ART) can produce a pregnancy in a woman who has gone through menopause using the donor eggs of a fertile woman in her twenties or early thirties.

FACT: Adoption has become a riskier venture in light of recent court cases.

FACT: Managed care insurance policies are limiting options and opportunities for infertile couples.

PREFACE

Extraordinary Measures, Ordinary Families

I am the 43-year-old mother of an IVF (in vitro fertilization) daughter and co-owner of seven embryos in a hospital freezer awaiting a final decision. Welcome to parenthood in the twenty-first century.

My husband and I belong to the estimated 15% of American couples who seek fertility treatment each year. The standard definition of infertility is one year of unprotected intercourse without a resulting pregnancy. That amounts to 12 serious disappointments leading to some strange revelations about our bodies. When we finally turn to the medical profession for treatment, precious time has elapsed. Our private wish to have a baby becomes a medical undertaking with all the public anxieties and costs that hospital procedures entail. In order to become an ordinary family, we must go to extraordinary lengths with no guarantee of the outcome.

In our case the process took 10 medicated cycles, three in vitro attempts, plus two transfers of frozen embryos. After much investigation and a few wrong turns, the final diagnosis was a simple fact: My tubes were blocked. I was 34 years old and an excellent candidate for in vitro. After five (five!) years of treatment I gave birth to a healthy seven-pound six-ounce daughter in 1992.

Gestation Fright to Gestation Frenzy

Emotionally I have traveled light-years since I published a magazine article in the early 1980s entitled "Gestation Fright: The Fear of Pregnancy."

With all the arrogance of a presumably fertile woman of twenty-something I described my hesitation about the process of childbearing. My fears ranged from the banality of gaining weight for nine months to the more profound issue, however remote, of death. After the pressures of college and graduate work blazing a career path required total focus. Although I got married in my twenties, I wasn't convinced that having a family was right for me.

So I moved into my thirties childless by choice. After almost 10 years of marriage no one dared ask me when I was going to have a baby. I made it crystal clear that family building was not a personal goal for us. But as my close friends began to have children, I decided to stop using birth control. Then I began to research a story for a leading women's magazine about how fertility drugs produced quintuplets for the Frustaci family. I learned that the definition of infertility is 12 unprotected cycles with no resulting pregnancy. In looking back at my calendar, I realized that we had exceeded that measure. Slowly it dawned on me that we had a problem.

I didn't have to look far to find another long-married couple in the same predicament. After all the precautions, the questions about whether the time was right for a baby, after both partners were in agreement on the issue, to find that the decision wasn't up to us was unnerving. The day that I forgot to check the results on yet another ovulation test and left it sitting in the bathroom all day I knew it was time to move on to a more aggressive course of action. The other couple recommended their fertility doctor, and I made the appointment for the next available slot, which was four weeks away. Maybe this will be our lucky month, I thought, with the fervent hope of a typical fertility patient.

Meanwhile the other couple dropped out of treatment. While the majority of patients are dedicated almost to the point of obsession, about 10% will opt out during the first year. The emotional and financial strains do take their toll eventually. For our friends, a child-free marriage was the right solution.

IVF Works! (Eventually, for Some of Us)

Over the course of 15 medicated cycles (plus 48 natural ones) I promised myself I wouldn't be greedy: If I could produce only one child, I wouldn't press for more. Of course, with in vitro there is a one in 10 chance to conceive twins (my daughter was one of four embryos transferred together). What fertility patient doesn't pray for the blessing of two for the price of one? Since my husband and I share the same birthday, there was some appeal to the symmetry of joint birthdays. But with IVF statistics at the time showing take-home-baby rates of under 15% for women between 35 and 39, I was aiming only for a singleton. Nowadays only-children are no longer the exception, thank goodness, the result of a combination of the infertile population and economic pressures.

Amazingly I produced 25 eggs in a single cycle following the fertility drug therapy that preceded my third IVF procedure. For two weeks I had injected myself with Lupron, a drug primarily indicated for prostate cancer patients that suspends hormonal activity in women. In the second week my husband injected me with a cocktail of the powerful fertility drugs Pergonal and Metrodin. A single dose of human chorionic gonadotropin (hCG) set ovulation in motion. Early one morning my team of doctors vaginally retrieved the harvest of eggs in a twenty-minute O.R. procedure. After sitting overnight in a petri dish with my husband's sperm, 15 fertilized to become viable embryos.

Two days later four embryos were transferred into my uterus; none implanted. How could they with all the fertility drugs in my system? My ovaries had hyperstimulated, a common side effect of the hormone therapy. I was uncomfortable and crampy, and I firmly believed that my body was too stressed to support a pregnancy. My sense was that the odds would be better with the transfer of frozen embryos at a later date, when my uterine lining was in its natural state. My hunch paid off three months later.

Fertility Patients or Medical Pioneers?

What do you do with leftover embryos? With three or four embryos per transfer, I potentially have two more opportunities to get pregnant through IVF. (There is no possibility of conceiving naturally since my first IVF attempt ended in an ectopic pregnancy and the removal of my fallopian tubes.) Although the last batch of embryos thawed perfectly, the next one may not. But if it does, I have the option of requesting an embryo biopsy, a new process that indicates the health profile of the cells. I could find out the sex if I so desired.

A 48-year-old mother of an IVF son with three frozen embryos in storage has decided to wait. Her husband, who has grown children from an earlier marriage, doesn't want another baby. "Maybe I'll wait until he's gone," she jokes. But with the strides being made in today's fertility technology it is no laughing matter. The truth is, this woman could give birth after menopause under certain circumstances.

During my long struggle to become a parent, I never considered this strangely luxurious scenario: two separate pregnancies for the price of one. Twins born on different dates. Of course, twins carried together are a possible outcome of the IVF procedure, a dream come true for many patients. What options are open to me and my husband? We could donate these embryos to another couple. Or to science. Or take our chances on another baby. Or discard them. In the brave new world of fertility technology couples are facing questions on lifestyle issues that they never imagined possible in those carefree days of birth control and recreational sex.

Birth control pills gave our generation the sense that we have control over our bodies and can plan our families to suit our personal agendas. Turn it off, turn it on through the miracle of modern medicine. Attend to career matters before you get into the business of growing a family is this generation's modus operandi. But there was one part of the equation we didn't consider: getting older.

Age is key to, maybe even the biggest factor in, the inevitable winding down of fertility. "I don't want to hear another fertility doctor call me old ever again," a 40-year-old caller told me with unbridled anger. A 40-

year-old man asked me if he and his wife could be tested to see how much longer they could postpone starting a family without missing out altogether. The fact that we have no control over our reproductive organs comes as a revelation to many couples. At age 37 I asked my doctor, an eminent fertility specialist, "Is my age a problem?" His answer branded itself in my memory: "Yes, but it's not an actionable one." Meaning there was nothing he could do about it.

Current scientific wisdom holds age 35 as the turning point in the business of making babies. All the medical strides in the world cannot change the quality of the basic materials required for viable embryos and take-home babies. Statistics show a slippery slope in success rates from all the top fertility clinics for couples in their forties. The baby boom generation looks in the mirror, and the reflection confirms youth, energy, and athletic ability. What it doesn't show is what's going on inside.

When Did This Happen to Me?

You mean I was taking precautions all those years for nothing? Suddenly the fear of getting pregnant turns into the fear of never getting pregnant. The humiliation, letdown, bewilderment, and sense of uncertainty descend all at once. No, the precautions were not unnecessary. They served as an affirmation that you were not interested in starting a family at that time in your life. But the gamble you take is whether your body will be able to produce a baby once you decide you're ready. And if you discover that you need treatment, how far are you willing to go?

In my capacity as a hot line volunteer for Resolve, the infertility network, I have listened to the gamut of fertility problems for more than five years. Yet no matter how desperate the situation may sound to me, the typical caller harbors the belief that one day she will conceive naturally, at home and without medical intervention. I know how tough it is to let go of that belief; it took me two years. Until there is a definitive diagnosis, certainly there is no reason not to cling to this happy picture. With 20% of cases of infertile couples categorized as "unexplained," there is a significant population riding a monthly roller coaster of hope and despair. But learning to let go of that ideal picture of the two of you holding the positive at-home pregnancy test can mean getting into treatment sooner with better results.

The hard facts of fertility treatment with its drugs and low success rates may feel like a cold shower by contrast with the romantic decision to start a family. As a rule, fertility doctors urge aggressive action from the start. "I feel like they just want the business," one caller complained to me. Until a couple is absolutely convinced that there is no other alternative, resistance to surgical intervention seems to be the norm. That's why it took me five years to have my daughter, although my doctor recommended IVF from our first meeting.

Hope, however, does spring eternal. In the 10 years that I've been involved in the world of infertility, both as a patient and as a Resolve volunteer, I have seen how it prevails even under the bleakest of circumstances. Because no matter how long the odds, you have to believe that treatment will work in your case. And yes, I have met beautiful, healthy children born of "miracle" pregnancies both to women over 40 who insisted on treatment and to others who had failed in IVF treatment or other therapies and later conceived at home. So who's to say when it's time to quit?

The Secret to Success: Timely Treatment

What is the secret to success? Every caller I speak to on the Resolve hot line wants to know. No matter how dire the diagnosis, despite all the medical intervention, each person is looking for that simple answer, for that magical pill. While the dream of natural conception never goes away, it is far outweighed by the winding down of the biological clock after age 35. The real secret is *getting the right treatment for you right now*.

Unlike prior generations, we can turn to fertility clinics for help. Experts around the world are working on the key issues and introducing new procedures each year. From day to day the technology improves, which means that a greater number of the infertile are having families. In today's world a man can have one single sperm and manage to fertilize his wife's egg through micromanipulation in the laboratory. When I entered treatment in 1987, the field of cryopreservation had not yet been applied to the human population. By the time of my third IVF attempt at the end of 1991 it was a standard part of the fertility program I was enrolled with, and it was the method that produced my daughter. I could rationalize that delaying surgery worked in my favor since I benefited from the newest technology. The fact that I was under 40 with a clear-cut case of blocked tubes also contributed to my successful pregnancy.

Perseverance is the first ingredient in the secret of success. Staying the course means paying attention to the calendar, checking for ovulation in the short term and reflecting on how each passing birthday affects your reproductive organs in the big picture. You have to be convinced that biological parenthood is for you. The second ingredient of the secret is *pinning down your diagnosis*. This search may be a circuitous series of tests and retests to identify the problem area. It may entail seeking out specialists, reading medical journals, and learning more about your reproductive system than you ever bargained for. And the final variable is the doctor you choose to help you attain the goal. *Finding the specialist who is right for you* can mean the difference between a successful pregnancy this year or spinning your wheels for a series of cycles with no results.

The typical fertility patient aggressively researches the field and manages her treatment. Taking control of the treatment helps counterbalance the lack of control we have over our reproductive functions. Since the field is so new, and protocols tend to change from medicated cycle to medicated cycle, there is room for patient input. For example, I requested for my own comfort progesterone suppositories rather than the large-needle progesterone shots after my embryo transfers. Some of the clinic nurses expressed surprise at the doctor's compliance, and even I don't know how I got him to agree. Earlier in my treatment I opted to forgo the endometrial biopsy, which I'd heard was a painful and inconclusive test. Again, the doctor complied. He said we had sufficient evidence from the workup to conclude that my tubes weren't functioning.

But how the process tests your mettle! Who in her right mind looks forward to undergoing surgery, even if it may mean that her dearest wish will be realized? Each step of the way your commitment is challenged. If only I had a nickel for each time I heard someone extend her original parameters. "I would never do in vitro" becomes "I'll try it just once" and then "I'll give it one more chance."

And there are some heavy unknowns in the IVF process, not even for the babies as much as for the mothers.

Statistics show that the health profiles of these babies correlate to the population at large. For the mothers, however, it is too soon to measure what the long-term effects of the fertility drug therapy may be. Some doctors find a correlation between Pergonal or Clomid treatment and maternal ovarian cancer. Others say that the connection is unproved. Yet the question exists, and the fertility patient must consider potential risks.

Wake Up from the Nightmare

After suffering an ectopic pregnancy following my first in vitro attempt, I participated in a support group of women who had recently suffered lost pregnancies. One member of the group summed up the general feeling. "I just want my husband to kiss me," she confessed, "and say, 'Wake up, honey. Everything is going to be okay. It was just a bad dream.'"

Imagine the nightmare of undergoing the entire in vitro process, pumping yourself full of fertility drugs and finding that you're pregnant but that you won't be able to carry the baby to term because it's stuck in your tube. That's what happened to me with my first IVF pregnancy. Severe abdominal cramps turned my good news into a life-threatening situation. "Your life is in danger," the doctor warned me. "If that tube ruptures, you can bleed to death."

Prior to the termination the doctors couldn't guarantee that the surgery would be done through my belly button. The possibility of major abdominal surgery and the lengthy recovery that follows could not be ruled out, depending on the location of the embryo. I didn't sleep a wink that night, wondering how my happiest moment had turned around so hideously.

Keeping up a good attitude during treatment means banishing the thought that you may be one of those patients to lose a pregnancy. Didn't the doctor insert the embryos in the proper place for optimal growth? I found out the hard way that 6% of IVF patients experience tubal pregnancies. Since tubal disease is prevalent in this population, the chance that an embryo will implant in the scar tissue can't be ruled out. The good news was that I could get pregnant with IVF. The bad news was that I had to return to square one.

Perseverance, commitment, experienced specialists, and, most important, a supportive spouse got me through the worst of the fertility maze to the desired end. The solid base of a long-term marriage helps put the pursuit of a family in perspective. As you go through the motions at work and with your friends and family, you and your husband retreat to a private world of menstrual cycles, hypodermic needles, and countless doctor visits. Meanwhile it feels as if everyone around you were expecting, some for the second time. Every fertility patient knows the strain of keeping a smile plastered on her face at yet another baby shower. Why is it so easy for all these other women? And why is it so easy for those child abusers? Angry thoughts are hard to keep at bay.

In the early 1990s, when I was undergoing fertility treatment, the field was in a start-up mode. The selection of specialists was definitely limited, as were the treatments. No scandals had erupted in the press. Couples actively pursuing so-called test-tube babies were the exception. Without much choice, of course it was simpler to make decisions.

How far-reaching and widespread the issue has become since those days! In today's world I bump into people in fertility treatment wherever I go: from people at the bank or at a cocktail party to legal counsel to neighbors to business contacts I've worked with for years. Even if it's not a personal issue, it seems that everyone has a sister, friend, or cousin in treatment. The conversation starts the same way, with a question inquiring after my daughter. Once I reveal that thanks to the efforts of IVF, I am a proud parent, the questions start spilling out. Even the smallest nugget of information can be a boon when you're facing the brave new world of fertility treatment with limited resources and health coverage cutbacks.

To these intrepid parents-to-be I offer the latest-breaking answers from reliable medical sources to the questions most often asked of me. Use this book as a guide while you come to understand your body's foibles and the tricks that time plays on all of us. I have packed in practical information along with the technical in the hopes of making your journey a smoother one. With the pressure of time bearing down, this book is intended to make your research easier. You are not alone in this pursuit, although you may think that you are standing still while others are building their families.

From personal experience I urge you to take the shortcut where possible, not to regret the past, and to keep abreast of the strides that have been made in the laboratory. Maybe I'm a Girl Scout at heart, but instead of dwelling on "Why me?" I like to think of fertility treatment as part of my journey. Yes, there is a part of me that feels deserving of a badge for going through the process. But along the way my path crossed that of special people I wouldn't have otherwise met, including many eminent doctors and nurses. I appreciate my daughter with a healthy respect for modern medicine.

I wish you speed and success in your journey in the world of fertility. Good luck!

101 ANSWERS TO YOUR FERTILITY QUESTIONS

PART I

FACING THE FACT OF INFERTILITY

TEN MOST COMMONLY ASKED QUESTIONS

1. DIAGNOSIS: How do I know that fertility treatment is appropriate for us?

Doctors define infertility as the inability to conceive within the course of one year of unprotected intercourse for couples aged 35 and under. For couples over 35, six months of activity without birth control and no resulting pregnancy qualifies as a signal of a possible underlying condition. *Just because you get your period like clockwork does not mean that you are fertile or even that you are ovulating. Don't let that false hope lull you into putting off a consultation with your doctor.*

Other obvious signals of trouble include: irregular periods, one or more miscarriages, exposure to DES, and chronic health issues. If you fall into any of these categories, then it may be time to recruit medical help.

To maximize results on your own, use a calendar. Sexual relations should take place around the time of ovulation, which occurs 10 to 14 days following your last period. Experts agree that the key is to time intimacy to the release of a Graafian follicle (egg) from the ovary rather than to concentrate on frequency. If the egg doesn't combine with a sperm along the way at the appropriate time, it will be expelled by the body, and menstruation will take place about two weeks later.

Besides looking at the calendar, how do you know when you're ovulating? There are three ways you can gauge it yourself. One is by observing physical symptoms. A small number of women experience mittelschmerz, a twinge or cramp that signals ovarian activity about halfway through the cycle. Another simple method is to track your temperature for the first two weeks of your cycle. If you use a basal body (rectal) thermometer, leave it in a jar of petroleum jelly by the bed so that you can use it first thing. Record results every morning, beginning right after your last period ends. You'll experience a small surge (about half a degree) around the time of ovulation, although you must take into account a margin of error of a day or so.

Or you can invest in an ovulation kit, readily available at the local pharmacy for $25 to $65. (In 1996 *Consumer Reports* recommended the Clearplan Easy One-Step at under $30 if you have a regular cycle, the $65 OvuQUICK Self-Test if you do not.) Hormone levels in your urine show where you are in your cycle and help you coordinate intercourse for your most fertile day.

What is the most fertile day of the month? It's the day of ovulation, known as Day 14 for the woman who enjoys a regular 28-day cycle. Since sperm survives in the uterus for up to 48 hours, chances of capturing and fertilizing the egg are best *prior* to its release. Don't bother going overboard in the bedroom; sex every other day may work better in order to give sperm counts the opportunity to rebuild. Standing on your head or keeping your legs elevated can't hurt, although it's unlikely to change the course of events. Douching is absolutely a no-no.

Is it imperative to coordinate sex to the precise date of ovulation? Only if you haven't conceived over the course of several months. Chances are that conception will occur within a year (12 menstrual cycles) as long as all systems are in working order. The younger you are, the sooner you should achieve a pregnancy.

What if you're under 35, haven't conceived in six months, and are getting worried? Trust your instincts and speak to your gynecologist. Sometimes a sense that something is amiss is based on a real problem that can be either corrected or acknowledged and acted upon. With infertility becoming more prevalent among younger women, it's advisable to get a "workup" (fertility checkup) just to make sure that all the parts of the reproductive system are functioning properly. Specifically, a man needs to know that he is producing sperm that can travel (are motile), while a woman needs confirmation that she is ovulating, that her fallopian tubes are open, that the cervical mucus is a welcome environment to her partner's sperm, and that her uterus can carry a pregnancy.

If you leave for work before reading the results of your ovulation kit, the way I did the last time I invested in one, then it's definitely time to opt for a more aggressive course.

See: Ovulation, Postcoital test, Workup

2. RESPONSIBILITY: *Where does the fertility problem lie most often, with the man or the woman?*

Nature is very fair in the way it assigns responsibility in the universe of subfertility: Male factor (problems with sperm quality) accounts for a 40% share, female factor for another 40%, while the balance is equally divided between a combined couple problem and the frustrating catchall "unexplained." Once you have a diagnosis it will be expressed as a *factor* for which there is an appropriate course of medical treatment.

For men the central issue revolves around blockage of sperm ducts either as a result of a sexually transmitted disease (STD) or of a vasectomy or of the appearance of varicose veins in the scrotum. The most common female diagnosis (one in three) is tubal factor, often caused by complications following STD or PID (pelvic inflammatory disease). Ovulation factor ranks second, appearing in one of four patients. Remaining factors include uterine, cervical, and peritoneal factors, which may be connected to endometriosis.

Frequent press coverage on this subject gives the impression that infertility is on the rise in our country. In fact, statistics haven't changed on this front for more than 30 years. The National Center for Health Statistics estimates that since 1965 this medical issue has affected about 8.5% of the pool of potential parents in the United States. Why then is so much attention devoted to fertility these days? Because where nothing could be done before, treatment is now available to a wide cross section of this population. Unlike those childless friends of our mothers, our generation has the opportunity through medical intervention to carry one baby—or twins—to term.

What also differs from our parents' generation is the placement of family planning in the big picture. For our mothers, marriage and children came ahead of career. As we approach the millennium, two trends have come to light for the so-called baby boomers: (1) the postponement of parenthood until after age 35 and (2) a resurgence of venereal infections. Maybe toughest to digest is the issue of age: Couples in two-career families are choosing to wait longer to start families. At the risk of my sounding antifeminist, postponing pregnancy until after age 35 is a gamble with nature that must be weighed against career goals. Women are now facing the fact that the tradeoff for establishing careers in their twenties and thirties may entail investing some of their hard-won earnings in fertility treatment. Medical experts have strong scientific evidence that the late thirties are a slippery slope in the business of making babies.

Venereal infections, which have been on the increase following the introduction of the birth control pill, have also compromised fertility for both sexes. Gonorrhea, chlamydia, and syphilis all negatively impact on the fallopian tubes in the female partner and may damage the production and quality of sperm in the male. It is hoped that renewed use of condoms in the new sexual protocol to prevent the spread of AIDS will reverse the VD epidemic of recent years. Are marijuana and recreational drugs a factor? If smoking tobacco is suspected to compromise fertility, then it has to be considered that drugs of any sort may be a factor as well.

A definitive diagnosis often evokes a mixed reaction of relief with feelings of guilt in the partner who has the problem. While finding a reason for why conception hasn't occurred within your personal time frame offers a course of action, it puts pressure on the partner who requires treatment. Fortunately most clinics have full-time psychologists on staff to help couples deal with the emotional aspects of treatment. Rather than use the diagnosis as a license to assign blame, take advantage of it to pursue the appropriate treatment for your case. Don't look back; look ahead to the future.

3. FERTILITY SPECIALIST: How do I find the best fertility specialist in my area?

First, ask your gynecologist for referrals. If you both agree that your case merits a specialist, or at least a consultation with one, your current doctor can recommend a reproductive endocrinologist (RE) affiliated with the local hospital. The RE is an ob/gyn with an additional two years of training specifically in the field of fertility. For your husband, the first (and last) resource is his urologist. He should have a semen analysis before you go for a consultation with the reproductive endocrinologist. Don't wait until your examination. This way you will have the answer on whether there is a male factor in your case before you embark on further treatment.

Your second resource is other women. If you're like me, chances are you have bonded with at least one other woman who's taking medical action to get pregnant. I found my RE through a colleague of my husband's. Word of mouth is a reliable way to find help since you can find out more about how responsive the doctor is and what you can expect from the billing department. Some practices are willing to work with you with sensitivity to what your insurance carrier covers.

If you're the kind of person who's good at her homework, you can obtain a list of accredited specialists in your locale by contacting the American Society for Reproductive Medicine (ASRM) directly. Established in 1944, this association counts more than 10,000 members in its ranks. Among its subgroups is each specialty: the Society of Reproductive Endocrinologists (SRE), another for Reproductive Surgeons (SRS), and for Male Reproductive Urology (SMRU). Perhaps the most important service the ASRM provides is its publication known as the SART Report, the bible of fertility statistics, which appears every two years. Data from nearly 250 fertility clinics nationwide are compiled by the Society for Assisted Reproductive Technology (SART) affiliate. You may purchase the entire report for $90 or request a regional directory for $35. Because of the time required to collect and prepare the information, results are somewhat out-of-date by the time they appear. Yet it is a valuable source that can lead you to the right place for your diagnosis.

You can also find a local specialist through the volunteer fertility clearinghouse, Resolve. Its national hot line number in Boston—(617) 623-0744—can provide your local chapter telephone number. While it's helpful to know who is in the area, the type of coverage you have and the appropriate treatment for your case may guide your ultimate decision.

Finally, how do you evaluate a fertility doctor? This is a tricky issue since no government agency is setting standards or regulating the field at this time. Statistics are compiled and calculated differently from practice to practice in ways that may be confusing or, worse, misleading. Major fertility centers have been accused of overstating success rates. Even specialists admit that without any regulating body to set standards, unscrupulous reporting procedures do exist. The 1992 Wyden bill is attempting to correct this situation, a costly and time-consuming task. Sponsored by Senator Ron Wyden (Oregon), this legislation is attempting to set standards within the field of reproductive medicine. As "the Fertility Clinic Success Rate and Certification Act," the law was passed in 1992. However, due to lack of funding, it has yet to be implemented under the leadership of the Centers for Disease Control and Prevention. In the meanwhile the SART Report is attempting to set up uniform guidelines for calculating success rates.

How can you protect yourself and preserve your peace of mind as you embark on this expensive medical journey? Think of yourself as a partner entering an investment opportunity with all the attendant risks and rewards. Before you shell out your money, you need answers to five basic questions:

1. *Certification:* Is the doctor a board-certified RE or board-eligible (preparing to take final boards)?
2. *Outside auditor:* Has an outside auditor been retained to review the success rates of this practice? (Many groups are turning to well-known auditors such as Arthur Andersen for credibility.)
3. *Availability:* Is the office open 365 days a year? (You want to be assured that your treatment will not be compromised because of holidays.)
4. *Laboratory facilities:* Are full-time ultrasound and lab technicians on staff? Both are necessary once you begin fertility drug protocol and require close monitoring.
5. *SART membership:* Does the program belong to the SART registry? This is an important requirement since SART is setting the guidelines on these data.

With the trend in fertility treatment leaning toward group practices, the next step is to learn more about the personalities and policies of the program. For example, who will answer your telephone calls: the doctor or the nurse? The larger the fertility group, the more likely it is that a nurse will get back to you since she is much more accessible. While you may prefer to have your conversations with the doctor directly, you have to take into account the number of patients enrolled in the program and the fact that the doctor spends a considerable amount of time in the operating room. It may be in your better interest to select one nurse as your friendly contact when you have an urgent question.

Before you sign up, develop a plan of action with your husband. You will need some parameters, both emotional and financial. Determine together how many cycles you want to invest with this doctor. If you don't see results, or you think that your case is falling through the cracks at a busy office, move on. As a rule of thumb, if you don't see results within three medicated cycles (five, tops), consider switching to another doctor for a different perspective. But switching from doctor to doctor after a single cycle is ineffective and could indicate an unwillingness to accept an unfavorable diagnosis.

Time is of the essence in the pursuit of pregnancy, and you owe it to yourself to rise above the stress and disappointment factors to manage your case for best results.

See: Semen analysis, Workup, Ten Key Fertility Contacts

4. COSTS: *What is the average cost of fertility treatment?*

Just getting in the door costs between $200 and $400 for a consultation with a fertility specialist in the United States. Depending on the services you require, the range of charges spans from about $400 for insemination to $10,000 per cycle of in vitro fertilization or more if you require micromanipulation.

In countries with socialized medicine, each citizen is covered in the event of a fertility problem. Australia, for example, currently covers six in vitro attempts per lifetime. At the present time 2% of the Australian population is comprised of IVF babies. Health coverage for Americans is generally assigned through their employers. Where fertility treatment is concerned, some insurance policies cover little or nothing, while others set a limit on how many in vitro attempts are permitted. If you have only a single covered cycle, it is a big gamble since the odds of success on a first attempt are so low. The emotional cost may outweigh the potential benefit.

Efforts are under way to standardize this growing part of the medical industry in order to serve better the millions of people seeking help. Congress is considering the issue of preexisting conditions in order to allow for better portability of health coverage. Fertility clinics are trying to give credibility to the way success rates are presented by hiring third-party auditors to tabulate their results. But without national standards to regulate statistical reporting within the field, the medical consumer often has to bear the brunt financially to ensure successful treatment.

Right now the trend is to go for a procedure that is covered by insurance rather than one that will cost out of pocket even if the latter may be the more effective route. The issue of insurance becomes complicated when treatment adheres to what a carrier covers rather than what benefits the couple most directly. For example, in the case of tubal damage most policies cover repair surgery. The notion that the surgeon will fix your fallopian tubes so that you can go home and get pregnant sounds practical and sensible. Unfortunately, repair surgery has a low rate of success, and many of these patients may subsequently turn to in vitro anyway. But as long as the repair procedure continues to be covered, and people like me cling to a hope of natural conception, this extra, often needless step will continue to delay the inevitable.

5. INSURANCE: *Which type of insurance is best?*

Socialized medicine in countries like Australia and the United Kingdom seems to offer the best scenario for fertility treatment: Your taxes pay your way. Although statistics support the fact that infertility is a public health issue in the United States, underlined by the fact that the business of IVF now generates about $500 million a year, our country hasn't stepped up to bat on this subject. What's worse, the current trend of managed care may make treatment an even more expensive and elusive proposition for each couple.

This is one case where being an educated consumer may mean the difference between getting what you need or just getting in debt. As with all medical procedures, payment is required by the doctor at the time of service. Regardless of outcome, you will be charged. I have witnessed patients carrying briefcases of cash into the doctor's office and others charging treatment to their credit cards. I have spoken with people who told me how they put aside $5 a week until they accumulated enough money to pay for their next procedure. Despite efforts by the American Society for Reproductive Medicine, which officially recognized infertility as a disease in 1990, the insurance community continues to view its treatment as elective or experimental rather than required or standard. With so many people pursuing medical help to start families, how much longer can fertility procedures be considered experimental? As long as IVF—the technique that most defines the fertility industry—remains a high-cost, high tech procedure with low success rates, insurance companies will be reluctant to offer better coverage. Until the field standardizes or results improve, the resistance will be hard to wear down.

Generally, procedures leading up to IVF are covered to some degree while IVF itself (including the drug therapy) may be excluded. For example, if you have an ovarian cyst, you are covered for diagnostic tests and corrective surgery. However, if you need further medical intervention in order to achieve pregnancy, you may not be covered. In my case I was 80% covered for the IVF procedure in 1990. Yet when that pregnancy proved to be ectopic, I was 100% covered for the surgery to remove it.

What is the best way to approach insurance? Become a proactive consumer. Once you have a diagnosis, request a predetermination from the carrier. Become familiar with your policy, focusing on the section that describes exclusions, and look for loopholes if you need to. When no mention is made of a specific procedure you need, you have the opportunity to argue that it is covered by omission. If your carrier covers a diagnosis related to fertility, you may be able to make a case for follow-up treatment despite a denial. Don't despair if IVF isn't an approved procedure; break it down into the components. Find out if related tests (ultrasound, blood work, etc.) are covered, as is usually the case.

Work with your doctor's billing department on how charges are coded. If a claim is rejected as "experimental," resubmit the bill with a note from your doctor explaining the medical necessity for the procedure. Buy a special notebook and log all exchanges. A steady correspondence with a claims supervisor at your carrier may be an excellent investment in your future. At the very least you will have a clear record for tax purposes. Challenge any denial in writing; the telephone is not appropriate for the case you want to build. You deserve a full explanation for why the carrier made a decision. On your part, explain the medical justification for each claim that is denied by providing additional information. Seek out written statements from accredited organizations, such as the ASRM or the American College of Obstetricians and Gynecologists, that justify the medical value of your care and send it along.

The impact of the struggle between people seeking help and the insurance industry has affected which patients are accepted into some programs. Nowadays women 40 or over may find doctors reluctant to treat them unless they consider ovum donation from a younger woman. Limited coverage has also affected the way patients select specialists. If your carrier will reimburse only a single IVF attempt, obviously you will be concerned with a practice's success rates. Of the few hundred fertility programs nationwide, about two dozen are well known for good results. At this writing, these practices are being swamped by eager couples. Even those "lucky ones" who sign up with one of the well-known programs may face a waiting line of months—as much as one year—before they can be scheduled for treatment.

What about those IVF programs that guarantee a take-home baby or (most of) your money back? The fee for this package exceeds a nonguaranteed IVF within each practice, presumably as a premium. (Fertility drugs are extra and above the fee, adding another couple of thousand dollars to the cost.) No other medical specialty has dared risk such a promotional offer. The Society for Assisted Reproductive Technology (SART) Ethics Committee is scrambling to formulate guidelines. Meanwhile the American Medical Association has expressed disapproval of this sales approach as manipulative of the patient and potentially unethical for the doctor, who may go to unsafe lengths to avoid a refund. For example, one such program has been known to transfer 10 or more embryos per cycle (beyond the recommended maximum of four), which raises the odds of a multiple pregnancy. Since the money-back offer went into effect only in 1996, it's too early to measure results. Is it too good to be true? With eligibility limited to couples under 35, odds are stacked in favor of good success. (Couples over 40 may buy the package if they agree to accept donor eggs.) Just getting accepted into such a program implies you're an excellent candidate for IVF. At the very least it's a vote of confidence that may lift your spirits.

Once you are enrolled in a program, get all the estimated costs for your treatment in writing prior to each procedure. Calculate out-of-pocket expenses, such as travel or time out of work. Keep in mind that you may deduct medical expenses on your income taxes after they exceed 7.5% of your adjusted gross income.

If you have any extra energy, drop a line to your member of Congress, senator, or state insurance commissioner requesting that fertility treatment be mandated in your state. Legislation may require comprehensive fertility coverage for all residents (as in Massachusetts) or at least require carriers to offer employers the option of covering this disease. Currently a total of 12 states have enacted such mandates: Illinois and Ohio in the Midwest; Montana, California, and Hawaii out West; Massachusetts, Connecticut, New York, and Rhode Island on the East Coast; Maryland and Arkansas in the South; and Texas. Perhaps if fertility patients mobilized on the scale of the breast cancer lobby or Act Up (the AIDS advocacy organization), benefits packages would acknowledge this disease and ease the financial burden.

6. CANCER: Do fertility drugs cause cancer?

Not according to current studies. No sweeping cause and effect has been recognized to date between exposure to fertility drugs and subsequent development of breast or ovarian cancer. On the contrary, in cases where medication helps produce a take-home baby, fertility treatment may be staving off ovarian cancer for some women.

But it may be too soon to breathe a sigh of relief. Pergonal was introduced in 1967, Clomid in 1969. How their usage affects the long-term health of the first generation of women who have undergone fertility treatment remains to be determined by the year 1999, when two National Institutes of Health–funded studies are expected to be completed. After all, the negative repercussions of DES did not appear until it had been in use for nearly 30 years. The real impact of fertility drugs is also clouded by the fact that older women pursuing pregnancy may have reached an age when cancer becomes more prevalent. Did the drugs cause the cancer, or was the cancer a preexisting condition? The distinction may be difficult to draw. Resistance to fertility medication may indicate a higher risk. One 1996 study reported in *Fertility and Sterility* magazine inferred that women who do not respond to fertility treatment and have never given birth are more likely to develop ovarian cancer. The use of fertility drugs does not appear to contribute to a potential cancer risk by itself.

The basic drug protocol—pumping extra female hormones into your body to create artificially induced ovulation—would seem to impact on the female organs. Could the prolonged use of fertility drugs irritate the ovaries and increase a predisposition to ovarian cancer? One study from the early 1990s reported some evidence that continuous consecutive cycles of Clomid (the fertility pill) without an ensuing pregnancy may result in the development of ovarian tumors. While these results prompted doctors to prescribe Clomid less liberally, to no more than 12 cycles per individual, consensus on the subject is that research is still lacking.

One comprehensive fertility study, spanning almost 20 years, has been following 10,000 Australian women. Assumptions were made about this patient population on the basis of the average occurrence of cancers of the reproductive organs in the female population of Melbourne. Results were comparable for women who used fertility drugs and those who did not for cancer of the breast (one in 14) and ovaries (one in 94). Positively, the rate for cervical cancer was reduced by half as the result of early detection with regularly scheduled Pap smears required as part of the fertility protocol. On the downside, a higher than average incidence of uterine cancer was noted among patients with diagnoses of unexplained infertility. The potential to develop this form of cancer is greater where the diagnosis is unexplained infertility, which may imply a predisposition.

If your mother or sister has had cancer of a reproductive organ, discuss the implications in your case with your RE. Fear of the medications should not prevent you from pursuing treatment if they can help your outcome. The Reproductive Medicine Network of the National Institute of Child Health and Development recently launched an ongoing study of new treatments for infertility and their potential risks.

Final reports from three federally funded studies are expected to become available before 1999. Results from 10,000 cases culled from five national programs (New

York, Boston, Detroit, San Francisco, and Cleveland) are being tabulated under the leadership of Dr. Louis Brinton. In Seattle the Fred Hutchinson Research Center is examining records of 12,000 female infertility patients, while Dr. M. A. Rossing, who linked Clomid with ovarian cancer (*New England Journal of Medicine,* September 1994), is working on an update.

7. TWINS: *What are the odds of having twins if I take fertility drugs?*

Breathes there a couple in treatment who hasn't sighed over the romantic notion of two for the price of one? Twins banish forever the stigma of infertility. Since my husband and I share the same birthday, the symmetry of having twins had a special appeal. Women have spoken to me of how great it would be to build their family with a single pregnancy. But the reality of carrying two babies to term, the likelihood of a neonatal stay for the newborns, and the logistics of caring for them after birth, paint a different picture.

Current statistics set the odds of multiples quite high at one out of three IVF pregnancies, with twins accounting for 28% of the successful conceptions. Another 6% produce triplets, while 0.5% have quads. One fertility doctor calls multiple births the "scourge of IVF," and the consensus among specialists is that multiple births are a "suboptimal" response to treatment. The reason: the inherent complications in carrying more than one baby to term. Even when conceived under natural conditions, multiples are often born prematurely, some well before the optimal 40-week gestation period. While hospital neonatal wards are well equipped to handle premature newborns, it is a costly proposition. Recent estimates claim that assisted reproductive technology (ART) multiples account for more than three quarters of newborns in the neonatal units. For the parents, there's the added emotional stress of returning home empty-handed while their babies require a lengthy hospital stay.

Ideally, the goal of each ART procedure is one healthy baby per pregnancy without the use of fertility drugs. So-called natural (unmedicated) cycles may be offered as an option for selected younger women in some of the larger in vitro programs in order to create a singleton pregnancy. As treatment stands today, up to four embryos need to be transferred per cycle for the best results, and this enhances the possibility of twins. Although you may exercise the option of multifetal selective reduction to remove some of the embryos surgically, no one advocates this method as a standard practice. In 1996 the journal *Fertility and Sterility* reported another, perhaps more widely acceptable approach for patients on Pergonal that would occur prior to fertilization: transvaginal aspiration of extra follicles. With this technique the number of follicles are reduced at ovulation so that no more than three follicles over 14 mm are released from the ovary.

The American Society for Reproductive Medicine is committed to eliminating the potential for quadruplets, as well as containing the odds of triplets to below 2%. Clearly the push is on for researchers to come up with the formula that will reduce the prevalence of multiple births among the patients of ART by increasing the implantation rate so that fewer embryos need to be transferred.

8. HERBAL REMEDIES: Are there natural remedies that I can try before I go on medication?

Exploring every possible avenue that may enhance the possibility of conceiving is part of the process when you're dealing with infertility. My journey led me through crystals, meditation, hands-on healing, and affirmations and ended up in the operating room anyway. Other people in treatment have confided similar spiritual pursuits, from special prayers being said for them to filling their homes with international fertility symbols to pilgrimages to Lourdes or other religious shrines. As a friend of mine said once about picking up found pennies, we need all the luck we can find.

The desire to conceive naturally may stay with you throughout your course of treatment. While some alternative resources may help you cope, better keep in mind that infertility is a condition with a structural or chemical pathology that requires medical attention. This is not to say that modern science is the only solution, but rather that it is a miraculous option that enables today's couples to realize their dream to have families.

Did my foray into the world of natural healing help my situation? Yes, I believe it did, and that deep-seated belief was a comfort during stressful times in treatment. No widespread studies have measured their power, but certainly herbal remedies predate the introduction of assisted reproductive technology. In my experience, one remedy seemed to have a tonic effect. It is a Chinese herb known as dong quai, a derivative of carrots, which is prescribed for "female troubles." This herb, available at most health food stores, comes in tablet or liquid form. I drank a few droplets dissolved in a cup of hot water, which was completely flavorless, in place of morning coffee. Since research has shown that coffee may negatively impact fertility, the question is which factor worked in my favor: giving up caffeine or drinking dong quai? Can its properties really improve fertility?

If you believe in the power of the mind, as I do, then this method is worth a try. I used it in concert with in vitro to great result.

See: Unconventional Methods

9. SUCCESS RATES: *What are the odds that fertility treatment will work for us?*

For women under 40, as of the 1996 SART Report, about one in five with IVF and one in four with related assisted reproductive technology (ART) treatments. On the basis of 1994 data, official 1996 success rates stand at 21% for IVF, 28% for gamete intrafallopian transfer (GIFT), and 29% for zygote intrafallopian transfer (ZIFT). For women over 40, odds are about 9% or one in 10 with IVF. Donor egg results for older women are remarkable at 47%. Yet since 1994 the top two dozen clinics claim IVF success rates of 50% per cycle in women age 37 and under. Frozen embryos may boost the odds to 75% in some practices. Overall, you can expect anywhere from one to five treated cycles depending on your age and diagnosis.

More than 25,000 IVF babies have been born in the United States since the introduction of this procedure on our shores in 1981. Of all the American newborns in 1994, 6,300 resulted from IVF, 1,300 from GIFT and 300 ZIFT. For IVF, clearly the most popularly applied form of ART, this figure represents an improvement of 3% in its category over prior Society for ART (SART) statistics. Of the total live births for the combined categories, nearly two thirds are singletons (one baby) with twins representing 28%, triplets 6%, and quads (or more) 0.5%.

These results reflect the joint effort of SART and the Centers for Disease Control and Prevention (CDC) to establish a standard of measurement in the reporting of results. The Fertility Clinic Success Rate and Certification Act of 1992 assigned federal responsibility for regulating the 250 or so clinics to the CDC, which is actively formulating policy. Within the industry SART is developing guidelines for data reporting and lab accreditation in order to meet government criteria.

Thanks to the ongoing research of fertility specialists, the odds are inching upward annually. Every year new technology is introduced to help overcome various aspects of infertility. For me, success dovetailed with the development of frozen embryo transfers with IVF in the early 1990s. More recently sperm quality has been removed as a roadblock because of the growing use of intracytoplasmic sperm injection (ICSI) in IVF clinics. Some experts consider this new treatment for severe male infertility on a par with the IVF revolution. Current research is focusing on enhancing embryo development through various methods: by eliminating fertility drugs, adjusting the culture medium used in the petri dish for improved IVF results, and investigating immunological issues, such as microorganisms that may negatively impact on implantation of viable embryos.

Provided that your individual treatment is based on an accurate diagnosis followed by appropriate treatment scheduled in a timely manner, you will get pregnant. For example, if tests prove that the only factor preventing pregnancy is tubal damage, then you can pursue in vitro fertilization (IVF) with every good hope no matter how old you are. If you are over 40, the option of the donor egg will boost your prognosis. Where there is a male factor, ICSI may offer a solution.

And if 12 or more embryos develop in a single cycle, according to some specialists, the odds are with you.

Once you pass 40, however, success is more elusive. The odds of conceiving may drop as low as 6% except when you use the donor egg of a younger woman. In that case, results shoot up to near 50% or better. In fact, most programs urge older women to opt for donor eggs for best results. (Another seldom offered option is to "scramble" your eggs with those of a donor to enhance pregnancy potential. This is not an optimal approach due to the duplicated preparations required for the eggs of the donor and the recipient.) Sperm quality is no longer a factor, as mentioned elsewhere, thanks to the ICSI revolution of injecting a single sperm directly into the egg. And since your uterus can be hormonally adjusted to restore its youthful level, it only remains to add a viable egg to the equation in order to create a pregnancy.

See: ICSI (intracytoplasmic sperm injection)

10. STRESS: Now that I'm in treatment, how do I cope with the stress?

Once the profound sense of disappointment subsides and you are ready to face medical intervention, it may help to acquire some relaxation techniques to help you get through each cycle. No matter how strongly you subscribe to the power of positive thinking, which plays an important role in staying with this process, you will face moments of anxiety along the way. The prescription to dispelling these negative feelings? According to current research at the Mind-Body Program for Infertility at the Harvard Medical School, it is learning behavioral management techniques, such as meditation and imagery. Whether you sign up with a support group or seek individual counseling from a trained therapist, you stand to benefit in the management of your treatment by learning how to dispel anxiety.

Under the leadership of Dr. Alice Domar, the Harvard study began in 1990 as a 10-week program of stress reduction classes. Six months after graduation, one third of the women had conceived. While these results are encouraging, the research has no control group to use as a comparative. (Too few patients were willing to forgo treatment in order to serve as the control aspect of the study.) Would results be the same without the benefit of this program? Possibly. But even those participants who did not get pregnant learned valuable lessons in managing anxiety, anger, and depression both in fertility treatment and in general. Dr. Domar's goal is to help patients reconnect with the joys in life, of which motherhood is a single aspect.

Dr. Domar has observed that the stress factor rather than a poor medical outlook discourages good candidates from pursuing treatment. No question about it, as with any worthwhile pursuit, there will be ups and downs. And the downs can go pretty low. You may be able to regain control of your feelings by incorporating 15 minutes of mental exercises in your daily routine. The exercise may be as simple as sitting quietly at your desk with your eyes closed and taking a series of deep breaths. Meditation is a powerful tool that has been shown to lower blood pressure and regulate heart rate. Audiotapes are available at your local bookstore to help you get into the mood. Practicing yoga at this time may be a welcome diversion with many immediate benefits.

Imagery was a great comfort for me. I actually clipped a photo of a mother and baby out of the newspaper, superimposed my face over the other woman's, and taped it inside my closet. Seeing myself as a mother worked as a visual affirmation of my ultimate goal. I also created a mental summertime "picture" of my husband carrying our baby at the shore of a nearby lake. Realizing this desired image has been one of the most satisfying achievements of my life.

In order to reach this level of control, I read widely from the New Age literature of Shakti Gawain and Louise Hay, among others, and joined a healing group that met weekly for years. The agenda of the group was to offer support to the members, each of whom had a different issue, ranging from AIDS to midlife crisis. Reaching out to others in need during your time of crisis helps you maintain perspective and appreciate what you have during the rough patches. Our group leader, a trained therapist struggling with infertility herself, led us through a tremendous journey of self-enlightenment. Need I add that this amazing lady ended up producing a "miracle baby" after quitting fertility treatment at the age of 40?

Another source of comfort is prayer, whether in a religious setting or not. For followers of Gawain and Hay, the solace of affirmations may supply the emotional balm. These are a form of prayer that give words to the images as you would like them to be. What kind of crackpot would sign up with a healing group and read up on New Age thinkers? you may wonder. A working woman in her mid-thirties balancing a career with a marriage of 10 years while tending to an ailing parent. Sound familiar? Fertility treatment will reintroduce you to the spiritual side of life. I have spoken with couples who have tried everything short of voodoo to try to influence the unknown forces to make this dream come true.

For me, the epiphany came when I read the title of the bestseller *When Bad Things Happen to Good Peo-*

ple. Even before I cracked the book open, it occurred to me that the lesson to learn is that bad things happen to everybody although we expect them to happen only to bad people. Certainly, it's not fair when bad things happen to someone like you or me who's followed the rules. But who said life was fair? Don't dwell on how you got here. Just accept your path, and be grateful that medical science has developed methods to help us through this part of the journey to parenthood.

SAMPLE AFFIRMATION

I am the picture of a healthy pregnancy.

Disease has no place in me, and I carefully guard my thoughts to nourish my embryo's development and prevent false ideas from gaining a foothold in my consciousness. My embryo and I are healthy and perfect.

I see myself as the perfect picture of life, successfully carrying new life unfettered by former thoughts of ill health. I am conscious of a perfect functioning in every part of my body working now to keep the embryo growing and comfortable in my womb, down to the tiniest cell.

Blessings upon my body and the embryo now residing and growing within, and I know that all is acting in accordance with divine intent. Blessings upon our family.

I release these thoughts with love, faith, trust, and courage. So be it and so it is.

TEN FALLACIES ABOUT FERTILITY: MYTHS AND MISCONCEPTIONS

11. MENSTRUATION MEANS FERTILITY: As long as I get my period, doesn't that mean I'm fertile?

No, not if you're over 35, and not necessarily even if you are younger. Getting your period every month is not the measure of fertility; your age and the condition of your eggs and reproductive system are. What your period proves is that you haven't reached menopause, but that doesn't preclude the possibility that you are perimenopausal (approaching menopause). Menstruating implies that you are ovulating, but that is not always the case. Even if your ovaries are releasing a healthy egg every month, your hormone levels may not be able to support a pregnancy.

Mistaking your period for proof that you are fertile may be the most expensive assumption you'll ever make. Yet it is a commonly held notion. A newlywed 45-year-old woman told me, "My husband and I want to wait a year before starting a family." Another woman of 48 decided to begin trying only at her last birthday, when her periods became irregular and made her think that she'd better go for it. The first revelation about the reality of postponing motherhood came for both women when the doctor introduced the subject of donor egg. With today's technology donor egg recipients can choose to carry a pregnancy even after menopause, and that further strips your period of any significance.

If only menstruation were a yardstick! Yes, your first period marks the beginning of your childbearing years. But since that momentous date you must factor in the natural wear and tear of the decades, which take their toll on your reproductive organs, as on all other parts of the body. Ovulation becomes less predictable despite the presence of a period, and the quality of the egg is less viable. What's more, each passing year allows opportunistic infections or conditions like endometriosis to damage the fallopian tubes. With venereal disease on the rise—nearly 1,000,000 combined cases of chlamydia and gonorrhea were reported in the United States in 1995—the chances of conceiving at home are reduced.

If your period is meaningless, what do you need in order to conceive the old-fashioned way? The female partner needs four basic physical elements: (1) *ovaries:* at least one working ovary with the ability to release a mature, healthy egg; (2) *tubes:* at least one that connects the ovary to the uterus to allow the egg passage; (3) *cervical mucus:* friendly and navigable mucus that allows the sperm movement toward the egg; and (4) *a healthy uterus:* one complete with a thick endometrial lining that can support the fertilized egg through a full-term pregnancy. The male partner has to contribute one sperm, preferably healthy and vital, although with ICSI medical science can work wonders.

What is the best age to start your family? Today's specialists recommend that you begin as early as possible, preferably before age 35. Aristotle, the ancient Greek philosopher, advised couples to begin a family at age 18 for the woman and 37 for the man. Why the disparity in age? Both partners would then reach the end of their fertile years at the same time, he reasoned.

Ancient wisdom measured fertility through simple at-home methods like having a young woman sit on a clove of garlic. If the odor of garlic was detectable on her breath, that was proof that her tubes were free and clear! If the tubes were believed to be blocked, the patient would be treated with an herbal douche. As for men, hot semen was believed to be most potent, most effectively ejaculated from a short penis before it cooled off. (The opposite is true, according to modern medicine.) After intercourse women were advised to cross their legs immediately. Some home remedies never change!

12. FERTILE GENES: *My mom was the original Fertile Myrtle, and I come from a family of six, so why should I be concerned about fertility?*

Fertility is not a genetic trait like physical features or a predisposition for certain diseases like cancer. Too often people in treatment look to celebrity mothers who gave birth after 40 as role models. You can't make assumptions about your case based on what you hear about another woman's history, even if she's your mother. Each case carries its individual set of variables, even from one pregnancy to another within the same couple.

The bottom line is that fertility peaks before age 35 and will begin winding down as a woman approaches menopause no matter how well she ages on the outside. According to Dr. Alan Berkeley, director of the NYU Fertility Program, around the 44th birthday success rates for patients in his care fall off sharply. While he acknowledges that each practice has documented successes for the over 40 crowd, these happy stories are the exception, not the rule.

Many couples derive a false sense of security from the fact that they were conceived by older couples. But there are no guarantees in the universe of reproduction, especially in the age of birth control. Recurrent bacterial infections or tubal scarring may mean impaired fertility for women, while men are facing diminished sperm counts. The whole issue of the biological clock came to light for working women who put career building ahead of family planning. That ticking may become a costly and frustrating undertaking later on. What you may inherit from Mom is early menopause.

Timing is a tricky issue and a personal decision. Just keep in mind that after age 35 for the average couple conceiving at home becomes a gamble. It's true that some older couples conceive easily and without intervention. Yes, we're fortunate that medical science is working to help couples produce a biological child when nature makes it impossible. As long as you make an educated decision now you will understand the consequences you may face later.

13. SECONDARY INFERTILITY: *I conceived my first child in just a few months, so why is it taking forever with my next one?*

About 1.5 million or more families may be struggling with conditions that delay the conception of a second or third child. The National Center for Health Statistics estimates that more than 50% of women having trouble conceiving or keeping a pregnancy have given birth successfully before. What causes your body to play this cruel trick? Most commonly, a symptomless infection may have scarred your fallopian tubes or perhaps you had a difficult delivery with your first child. Occasionally, scar tissue may form following a cesarean section delivery and leave behind a condition known as Asherman's syndrome. Or perhaps your husband's sperm is not what it was. Latent fertility problems may have developed over time. All the same syndromes that appear in couples with primary infertility can strike those with secondary infertility.

But unlike couples with primary fertility, families with secondary infertility are reluctant to pursue medical help. After all, the thinking follows that if you got pregnant naturally once, you can do it again. I have spoken with parents of school-age children who are still hopeful of conceiving after 10 years or more. Holding on to the picture of the "ideal" family with two parents and two children, considered a birthright by most couples, persists over time. Mothers have confided that they want to produce siblings for the sake of their only children no matter how long it takes.

How is the psychic energy invested in this picture affecting the existing child and family life in general? According to therapist Dr. Harriet Simons, a lingering depression may take its toll. The loss of control of both the reproductive process and the spacing of siblings may come as a huge emotional shock. Especially as other couples go on to increase their families as planned, the issue is difficult to avoid. Not a day passes that I do not face the question posed to me by strangers as well as acquaintances: When will you have another? While only-child families are more common, they are still far from the accepted norm.

As with all fertility treatments, the onus is on you to take action as soon as you recognize a potential problem. Statistics show that success rates with secondary fertility patients in treatment are better than the average for primary cases. The encouraging news is that there is

help to be had if you are willing to enroll in a progr...
Give yourself time to digest what is happening, and ac...
knowledge that it's painful.

14. REVERSAL OF TUBAL LIGATION: *What's the big deal about untying my tubes? I had my tubes tied after the birth of my second child. Now I'm remarried, my spouse wants a biological child, and I've agreed to reopen my tubes.*

Undoing this action is not as simple as it sounds. Fallopian tubes are not like faucets that get turned on and off with a flick of the wrist. The success of the reversal depends on which *part* of the tube was closed off. The best scenario is if rings or clips were used in the ligation. In that case the surgeon created a loop at the proximal end of the tubes that closed off entry to the uterus. Removal of the rings results in pregnancy rates of 50% or better. On the downside, the risk of a tubal pregnancy is increased because of the scar tissue inherent to such surgery.

For women whose tubes were cut or cauterized, reconstructive surgery is a dicey proposition. Your tubes will be checked by X ray to determine whether reconnection is possible, how extensive the residual scar tissue may be as a result of the ligation, and if the fringe-like protrusions by the ovary (the fimbriae) are functioning properly. As the damage moves away from the uterus, the less likely repair will work for you. At the farthest end of the spectrum, damaged fimbriae may create a hopeless situation. Just locating an experienced surgeon who specializes in this type of microsurgery may also require extra research. The key word here is *microsurgery* since major surgery (laparotomy, or a lengthwise incision down the abdomen) for this type of procedure is no longer widely recommended.

de to pursue the repair route, it's ad-
e how success rates measure against
ists training to perform more popular
as in vitro, reversal operations have
become outda___. As a result, the prognosis with IVF
may be more hopeful. While conceiving at home is always preferred, especially since you've done it before,
as long as you're going into the operating room, you
might as well maximize the chance for success.

Where vasectomy reversal is concerned, the procedure is simpler and infinitely more successful. To create
sterility artificially, the vasectomy disconnects or ob-
structs the vas deferens or epididymis. While the sensa-
tion of orgasm remains intact, sperm is removed from
the ejaculate and absorbed into the body. To reinstate
fertility, the surgeon performs a vasovasostomy or
vasoepididymostomy. Under general anesthesia, an incision is made in the scrotal area and the repair is made.
The patient may convalesce for about a week. According to a 1997 report from the New York Hospital-
Cornell Medical Center and the Population Council,
this procedure has a "delivery" rate of one in two versus one in three with intracytoplasmic sperm injection
(ICSI). In addition to better success, reversal eliminates
drug therapy for the female and the potential for multiple births.

15. CULTIVATING SPERM COUNT: *Does eating oys-
ters (or any other exotic food) help build a man's
sperm count?*

To date there is no evidence that oysters influence
sperm count. But if you are the very beginning of your
quest for a baby, you may want to turn to vitamin sup-
plements for optimal sperm production. Specifically,
three grams a day of an amino acid called L-carnitine

has been shown to improve both motility and count. The journal *Fertility and Sterility* reports that vitamin E therapy may also boost male fertility.

If your test shows a low sperm count, megadoses of zinc may help. One study boasted a 75% success rate with a sample of 101 men who took 440 mg of zinc sulfate daily for eight weeks. A 250 mg tablet of vitamin C every day has also been recognized to have valuable properties in diminishing oxidative sperm damage.

By the way, it has been proved that smoking, alcohol, and drugs take their toll on sperm. The good news is that sperm regenerate every three months. So a 90-day "dry-out" period for a man should ensure a good supply of healthy sperm.

16. EFFECTS OF TENSION: *"How can you get pregnant when you're so wound up?"* . . . *"Why don't you adopt? A child will put your mind at ease so that you'll conceive naturally."*

When your mind is set on having a baby, nothing is more irritating than to hear the word *relax*. What is less relaxing than to make your sex life public and have nothing to show for it? Just coming to grips with the concept of fertility treatment is enough to set your teeth on edge. If any remark is bound to raise your blood pressure, it's this one. Usually by the time you've reached out for emotional support or medical help on this issue, many fruitless cycles have passed. You're just beginning to wonder why you ever used birth control. Until you get to the bottom of why you're not getting pregnant, kicking back and smelling the roses just makes no sense.

Sure, there is physical evidence that when you're tense, you can throw your hormones off course. But after six months or so of unprotected intercourse have passed without a pregnancy, you have every good reason to take action and look into the matter more closely with the help of a specialist. As the realization hits you that you may not be able to conceive naturally, you're bound to go through a wide range of emotions. Rather than isolate tension as the obstacle to getting pregnant, approach it as a side effect. Certainly, developing avenues for releasing tension will be helpful in both treatment and outside. Meditation or yoga classes can help you summon the strength and focus that will carry you through this unexpected chapter of your life. If your doctor thinks that stress is a factor in your diagnosis, you can arrange for short-term counseling to alleviate symptoms.

Educating yourself about your diagnosis and treatment is another way to dissipate the tension of the waiting game. If you find that you manifest stress by suppressing ovulation and skipping a period, your diagnosis will help you into the right course of treatment. Just understanding what is going on inside your body may help after months of being in the dark. I always felt like a graduate student working with eminent medical pioneers on a mission to solve a major mystery, which happened to reside in my reproductive organs.

Dr. Alice Domar of Harvard has developed a stress relief program specifically tailored for fertility patients that has been shown to enhance the odds of conceiving. Success rates improve for participants in this program because they are willing to take a deep breath, learn how to deal with the attendant stress, and continue with treatment. Learning how to manage the stress involved in signing up to be a pioneer in the field of reproductive medicine helps you stay the course. But the bottom line to success is proper treatment. You need to identify what concrete, physical problem is holding you back from achieving your life plan.

When relaxing doesn't prove itself a tonic, well-wishers offer the adoption alternative. The implication here is that you're so wound up about becoming a mother that simply holding a baby will do the trick. Who among us hasn't indulged in this kind of magical thinking that an outside action—some kind of talisman, like a lucky charm or item of clothing—will influence the internal workings of our bodies? Who's to say that it won't? To quote a wise man (my husband), any flea powder that works is good flea powder.

Of couples coping with infertility who don't enlist medical intervention, research shows that about 5% will achieve pregnancy within the second year of unprotected intercourse whether they adopt or not. (The timing of the adoption, not the act itself, gives the illusion that it influenced natural conception.) Certainly, it offers one avenue to parenthood complete with its own set of anxieties and issues. But studies confirm that it is no guarantee of a "cure" to a structural defect or medical issue.

17. BIOLOGICAL CLOCK: *Don't men have to worry about their biological clocks? Is there an equivalent to menopause?*

Men are not exempted from getting older. Although menopause per se doesn't draw the line for men as it does for women at age 50, male hormone production does slow down over time. And the sperm of a 50-plus man may not be as viable because of reduced motility (speed) or hampered morphology (shape). Physical changes become noticeable in the genitals as the testes shrink and soften and as testosterone levels wane. Consequently, the sex drive may drop off and further complicate the pursuit of pregnancy.

Secondly, over the course of time chronic health conditions may arise that may affect the production of sperm. Medications may negatively affect the level of fertility. Then there is the wear and tear of adult habits. A lifetime of drinking or smoking may take its toll, and there is more opportunity for infection to strike. Childhood diseases, such as mumps or chicken pox, curtail fertility when they are contracted by a grown man. To protect yourself, it is advisable to know whether you had these illnesses as a child or if you need to be vaccinated.

Yet there is no age cutoff for men who pursue biological fatherhood after age 50, as proved by the septuagenarian actors Tony Randall and Anthony Quinn. As long as the female partner is under 35, the odds for success are high. Even where male sexual function is an issue, pregnancy can be achieved through insemination. And through the application of ICSI together with IVF, sperm quality is no longer an obstacle either.

See: ICSI

18. TIMING: What's the big rush about starting a family?

Indeed you do have all the time you need—as long as you recognize that the longer you delay childbearing, the more likely it is that you may require medical intervention in order to achieve your family. And after age 43, without donor eggs, there is only a slim chance of a biological baby. As you may be observing the hard way, the biological clock is a fact of life. Over time, particularly past age 35, the less viable your eggs will be to become embryos that turn into take-home babies. Despite the efforts of the best fertility doctor, you need to produce good-quality eggs to make a pregnancy.

The keys to success in the fertility business are *age* and *genetics*. As long as you are under 35 and not a known carrier of any hereditary anomaly, your outlook is excellent. Once you are 36 or older, the chances of chromosomal abnormalities appearing in your eggs are more likely for unknown reasons. The higher incidence of abnormal eggs triggers hormonal changes in your body as you approach 40. After 40 as a rule one in three eggs will be defective, and at 43 half are of poor quality. Yes, there are exceptions in the over 40 population, and you may fall into this fortunate category. Since follicle-stimulating hormone (FSH) levels fluctuate from month to month, you may be able to retrieve a sufficient number of viable eggs that will combine with sperm to create embryos. Yet for the majority of forty-ish women, fertility is on the wane as menopause looms ahead.

I am endlessly astonished by the power of denial about the inevitability of menopause. In fact, I have heard of a case where a woman hit menopause following her final (unsuccessful) fertility treatment at age 47. Women speak wistfully about how their grandmothers had "change of life" babies. But a late pregnancy is not a hereditary trait. Yes, it has happened and may happen to you. I have even learned of such a happy surprise recently, but the odds are stacked against you.

While this news is discouraging, there is an excellent opportunity for the 40-plus woman who is willing to accept a donor egg. Fertility programs are showing great success with the combination of a young woman's egg with your partner's sperm. You will be matched with a donor who resembles you and provided with her medical profile. Of course adoption is another good option.

Family building is certainly available to you at any age—as long as you are open-minded to the new technologies that you may require.

19. EXERCISE: Can too much or too little physical activity affect my reproductive organs?

When you begin to feel desperate about getting pregnant, you start examining everything you do under a microscope.

Every action becomes suspect, although there is no evidence that exertion impedes conception. Indeed, the same fertility factors (PID, endometriosis, miscarriage) affect women in every weight class except for one factor: ovulation. Extremes in weight may harm the natural course of ovulation. Underweight women may not be producing sufficient female hormones, while for overweight women the common suspects are hypertension and thyroid or adrenal gland conditions. Competitive athletes may keep body fat so low as to suppress ovulation. Even for the average woman any sudden shift in weight may affect hormone production and interfere with ovulation. Unless you are seriously overweight, put that diet on hold while you're in treatment.

Monthly periods do not guarantee that ovulation is taking place, and the doctor may test the overweight patient for Stein-Leventhal syndrome (aka polycystic ovarian syndrome or PCOS). Overweight is a symptom in only half of this patient population. Another common symptom of this problem is small, benign cysts beneath the ovarian surface that may be interfering with proper ovulation. In eight of 10 cases a prescription for Clomid will ensure proper ovulation. Half of these women will conceive naturally. When surgery is indicated, the prognosis becomes cloudy since excess weight may lead to complications (blood clots, infections, improper healing).

From personal experience I can report that I undertook a strenuous three-mile hike without adverse effect the day before receiving good news of a successful embryo transfer. (What I shouldn't share with you is the fact that since I felt crampy and pessimistic about the pregnancy test, I decided rather dramatically not to deprive myself of a day in the great outdoors.)

In the "olden days" of the 1980s the Mayo Clinic used to prescribe four days in bed following embryo transfer. That meant no bathing, showers, or movement at all. Dr. Jamie Grifo of the NYU Medical Center reports a patient with a bad case of diarrhea who spent hours in the hospital bathroom following a transfer yet carried twins to term. Once embryo implantation takes place, physical activity seems to have no bearing on proper fetal development.

While regular exercise may be good for your mental health during the course of fertility treatment, don't go overboard. Daily training to an extreme degree may interrupt ovulation. With muscles co-opting the body's oxygen supply, your hormone production may be inhibited, and your periods will become less copious as a result. Until you conceive, it may be advisable to skip the marathon this year.

See: Anovulation, Polycystic ovarian syndrome

20. MEDICAL CONTROL: *Since the in vitro process is completely under a doctor's supervision, how can anything go wrong?*

After you have tried to get pregnant at home under natural circumstances with no success, the involvement of a professional specialist tends to raise your hopes.

What a relief it is to have the advice of an expert and throw away those basal body temperature (BBT) charts! For men, the pressure of performing on demand is over. Now they can make their contribution in a cup.

Initially, the temptation to lean on the doctor is overwhelming. But the fertility patient soon learns that being proactive means seeking out the appropriate medical treatment for an accurate diagnosis. You must educate yourself on the subject, continually managing your case since chances are you are enrolled with a busy practice. Set parameters for your doctor: If you don't see progress within three to five cycles, look elsewhere. Too often I've heard of women who allow years to go by under the treatment of a trusted doctor only to end up with a stack of medical bills and no baby.

Seven factors play into what may go awry in the IVF setting.

1. Endocrinological factors may not fall into place. Your hormones do not respond to fertility drug therapy, and the cycle is canceled.
2. A genetic imbalance may manifest itself. Your embryos display structural defects and receive low grades.
3. A hatching dysfunction may stop the proceedings. The sperm do not properly fertilize the eggs to make embryos.
4. Suboptimal culture in the petri dish conditions could interfere with proper embryo development. Your embryos are not structurally viable.
5. A suboptimal uterine environment may undermine success. Your embryos do not implant.
6. The transfer methodology may queer the deal. The embryos are not replaced properly into the uterus.

7. Or finally—horrors—you suspect mishandling. The laboratory makes a mistake, and you are the recipient of some other couple's genetic material.

Sometimes all goes well with the IVF process, yet no pregnancy develops, and this may be the most discouraging scenario of all. With a success rate of 21%, obviously, 79% of cases meet with disappointment. Why are so many good embryos lost? Research on this question is just in the early stage as of this writing, with the focus on antibodies and immunology. Rest assured that help is on the way.

See: Autoimmune syndromes

PART II

THE WORKUP

QUESTIONS ABOUT YOUR FERTILITY CHECKUP

21. WORKUP (FERTILITY EXAMINATION): What can I expect from the workup?

After more than six months of unprotected sexual activity have passed without a pregnancy, your doctor will want to evaluate your reproductive capacity as a couple. General health will be examined first, and each of you will be tested for hepatitis and AIDS.

In the course of the workup you will be examined individually and together to determine a diagnosis based on one or more fertility factors: male, tubal, ovulation, cervical, or peritoneal. If nothing emerges from these results, you will be categorized under "unexplained infertility (idiopathic)." At that point you may elect to have further tests to identify whether immunological issues or other bacteria may be preventing a full-term pregnancy.

For the male partner the workup is relatively straightforward: a semen analysis and a general physical to determine if there is a male factor preventing conception. For the female, a battery of tests will check whether her five fertility factors are in working order. Her workup begins with a focus on the two factors that combined account for the diagnosis in more than half of all fertility patients: the tubal and ovulation factors.

Once a factor is identified, you can finally proceed with the appropriate course of treatment.

If the couple passes these three tests, the investigation moves on to the next question: How is the chemistry between the two of you? A postcoital test will measure the cervical factor to determine if it is a welcome environment for the sperm. If the doctor has more questions about the condition of the woman's tubes and pelvic organs, the peritoneal factor will be examined with a laparoscopy. This ambulatory procedure, which takes place in an operating room, allows a scope to enter the body through the belly button for a scan of the peritoneum—the membrane that covers the pelvic organs—to check for adhesions or other abnormal growths. This final test finds endometriosis in one of three women without a prior diagnosis.

Are there any shortcuts in the workup process? One school of thought among specialists is that since most roads lead to in vitro, why not advance right away—particularly if you are approaching age 40. With health insurance covering fewer items, this attitude may also be the most cost-effective. However, for younger couples, the traditional workup is often preferable since simpler treatments may get good results without the risk of multiple births.

22. FERTILITY SPECIALIST FOR WOMEN (REPRODUCTIVE ENDOCRINOLOGIST): *What does a reproductive endocrinologist do?*

When you have a female problem, you consult a gynecologist. A gyn or ob/gyn (obstetrician/gynecologist) answers your questions about birth control, pregnancy, and general health issues. But when you have a fertility problem, you need a reproductive endocrinologist (RE). After six to 12 months of unprotected sexual intercourse have passed without a pregnancy, it's time to take this step. An RE is a specialist whose practice focuses solely on overcoming the difficulties of conceiving. He or she may also be a reproductive surgeon, or microsurgeon, able to perform corrective procedures through the use of laparoscopic techniques. Since time is essential when you want to build a family—whether because of your age or simply your personal agenda—you want to go to the expert without delay.

This relatively new specialty requires a two-year fellowship on some aspect of infertility upon successful completion of the ob/gyn program. Since getting certified is a lengthy process, practicing reproductive endocrinologists may be board-eligible, which means they have yet to take the boards although they are fully qualified. With oral or written exams scheduled almost two years after the clinical training is completed, the time lag is understandable. Per guidelines drawn up the American Society of Reproductive Medicine (ASRM), each RE is expected to supervise 20 egg retrievals annually.

Endocrinology is the study of hormones and their regulation in the body. Reproductive endocrinology focuses on all issues—hormonal, structural, and bacterial—that may interfere with natural conception. Since the RE treats only couples with fertility issues, he or she can more quickly draw conclusions based on the results of your workup. In the event that further tests are recommended, the RE has the facilities, skills, and expertise in the field to make the arrangements.

The key component to the package is the embryology department, which represents the success of any ART procedure you may require. You want to check the laboratory's success rate with freezing and thawing embryos, which should show at least a 50% survival rate, and you want to ask about its track record with preimplantation embryology. Although this part of your medical team is behind the scenes, these folks can influence the outcome of your case.

Especially for couples who may be feeling frustrated in their pursuit of pregnancy, one session with an RE may confirm your faith in the medical profession. Even if the RE doesn't tell you what you want to hear, you will find direction or a diagnosis that will help you move on with treatment and with your life.

By the time you sit down with an RE, you probably have a folder of test results. I had six months' worth of basal body temperature charts that my gynecologist had given me to track my temperature and sexual activity. This information gives the specialist some insight into ovulation patterns and the length of your cycle. Arrange for all results from your workup to be sent to the RE prior to your visit. Although you may have to repeat some tests, this history may be helpful in gearing up for treatment.

As a rule, your initial appointment will be scheduled at the end of a cycle so that if you choose to enroll in the program, you can return on the famous Day 3 for blood tests to measure your hormone (FSH and LH) levels. AIDS and hepatitis need to be ruled out before you go any farther. You can anticipate plenty of blood tests throughout the course of treatment. (I still have needle marks in the crooks of both elbows from the pints of blood that were drawn.)

For women who have experienced two or more miscarriages, the new subspecialty of reproductive immunology may be able to offer new hope. If the loss is not due to a chromosomal abnormality, and structural or hormonal problems are ruled out, the immune system becomes suspect. Medical research has discovered that immunological disorders within the uterus may cause the body to reject the fetus as a foreign object. Sometimes women may produce antibodies that prevent conception altogether. How do you know if you have an immune problem? Through yet another blood test.

If the workup from your gynecologist was incomplete, your RE will recommend a full workup. Even if you had a full workup, your RE may want to redo some tests to double-check results. In addition to blood work, the full workup includes: semen analysis, postcoital test (PCT), ultrasound exam of the uterus, and hysterosalpingogram (HSG). If a luteal phase defect is detected, an endometrial biopsy may be recommended just before your next period is due. A pregnancy test is required before you undergo the biopsy, just to be on the safe side. In most cases, the final and most invasive part of the workup is a laparoscopy—a surgical look-see into the pelvis with a scope to check for obstructions—which is also scheduled at the end of your cycle.

23. FERTILITY SPECIALIST FOR MEN (REPRODUCTIVE UROLOGIC SPECIALIST): *How can a reproductive urologist help us?*

Occasionally a woman will embark on fertility treatment and finish a complex workup before her partner goes for a semen analysis. This is an unfortunate sequence of events, particularly since a male factor accounts for an estimated four in 10 fertility problems. If the effort to seek medical help is initiated by the woman, as is the typical case, it's understandable that her workup takes place first.

What is the benefit of consulting a reproductive urologist? While your current urologist is qualified to help you get a sperm count or correct any physical problem, the specialist can evaluate the results and work with the sperm. A reproductive urologist is a medical doctor with extra training in anatomical issues like microsurgical repairs and membership in the newly formed Society for Male Reproduction and Urology, a branch of the ASRM. Through experience in the field, this specialist knows what to look for in terms of sperm motility (speed), morphology (shape), or the ability to fertilize. This expertise extends into the operating room and helps expedite treatment and eliminates the search for a surgeon. The work is supported by andrologists—Ph.D. lab technicians who work closely with embryologists on hormonal issues or preparing sperm for ART procedures.

Is there a single syndrome or condition most responsible for male factor? Yes, according to the observations of andrologists. Of 10 male patients, four will suffer from varicocele (a varicose vein in the scrotum). Any enlargement in the veins that lead out of the testicle may have a detrimental effect on sperm production. Depending on the extent of the swelling, this condition may be corrected surgically. An equal number of male patients will fall into the gray area of "unexplained" infertility. In this case the andrologist will take the exam to the next level of testing and determine whether an immunological factor may be present.

Of the balance, one in 20 patients exhibits a hormonal imbalance, while another 10% have sustained testicular damage as the result of infection, illness, or injury. Seemingly innocuous childhood illnesses, such as mumps or measles, may impair fertility when contracted by an adult male. Occasionally, congenital abnormalities will appear. Most common are hypospadia, which is characterized by the opening of the urethra appearing under rather than at the end of the penis, or

the complete absence of the vas deferens. Your andrologist will recommend the appropriate ART procedure
(intrauterine insemination [IUI] or IVF) best suited to
your case. Men with diabetes or prostate disorders will
be examined for retrograde ejaculation, which is characterized by seminal backwash into the bladder rather
than release out of the body. Finally, the doctor will
check for any silent bacterial infection, which is suspected to pass unnoticed in an estimated 15% of the
sexually active male population.

After assessing your full medical history—taking into
account exposure to chemicals on the job, what you eat
and drink, any drug use, or medications for chronic
conditions—the andrologist will make a recommenda-
tion tailor-made for your case.

MALE FACTORS

24. SEMEN ANALYSIS: What is semen? How important is volume? What about freezing it?

The instant that you suspect a fertility problem, get your husband's semen analyzed right away—even before you consult your gynecologist. Semen is the fluid ejaculate produced by your partner during an orgasm. In addition to sperm, it contains chemicals and fluid. Testing semen is a painless, noninvasive procedure that will quickly identify or rule out any male factor problems in your case.

The urologist will request a "sample" (the polite term for *ejaculate*), for which you will receive a special cup. For a more accurate reading, the sample should be produced after a brief period of abstinence of about three days but no more than seven. If the sample is collected too soon after the last ejaculation (within 24 hours), the amount of semen may be diminished. On the other hand, if too many days have elapsed, then the semen may contain "old" sperm with impaired motility. In any case, the doctor will request more than one sample over the course of treatment to obtain an accurate reading.

For your husband's sake, producing the sample at home may be more comfortable since he is expected to masturbate into the cup. "You haven't lived until you've had the thrill of carrying your husband's semen to the lab under your arm first thing in the morning," one woman told me. I have been in the waiting room of a laboratory where a non-English-speaking man in treatment had to be led into the bathroom by a technician for a nonverbal demonstration of what was expected.

Most facilities have a specially assigned room for this function, complete with appropriate reading material. The doctor can supply special condoms for this purpose, if you prefer, so that semen may be collected during intercourse. However, laboratories discourage their use since condoms may contaminate the sample with toxic substances.

Results of the analysis will be available within days. Most facilities have computerized systems—computer-assisted semen analysis (CASA)—that can provide an accurate portrait of this key factor. The lab will be looking at five aspects: (1) count (actual number of sperm in the sample); (2) motility (ability to navigate); (3) shape (percentage of normal); (4) both thickness and (5) volume of semen produced. Average volume ranges from one fifth of a teaspoon to a heaping spoonful. Anything less may indicate that there is not a sufficient supply of sperm reaching the cervix. As long as a minimum of 40% of the sample meets the normal parameters, all is well.

What if the sample shows a predominance of abnormally shaped sperm? As long as there are some normal ones, fertility may not be compromised. But if the count or motility is low, that may set off some red flags. The urologist will want to look further into possible hormonal imbalances (thyroid, pituitary, and male hormones) through a series of blood tests. Sometimes an imbalance in the male partner will respond well to a protocol of fertility drug therapy.

See: Male hormone issues

25. SPERM COUNT: What is the measure of a good or bad sperm count?

I have heard of more than one man who framed the results of a sperm count and displayed it on an office wall for all to see. Nothing is wrong with a man taking pride in his potency, but this is one case where it may not pay to advertise. While the count may sound astronomical, it takes only a single quick, normally shaped sperm to fertilize an egg. The key to success is speed; without motion, sperm won't get far despite the abundant output.

The average sperm count ranges widely from 20 million to 150 million per milliliter of semen. The measure depends on age, the duration of abstinence, and, possibly, the region you live in. According to the results of a 25-year study comparing East Coast and West, the highest sperm count in the United States is found in New York City, while Los Angelenos rank 50% below. The average sperm count in New York is 131 million, as compared with 101 million in Minnesota and 72 million in L.A. This study found no decline in either motility or volume over time. Location, location, location is taking on new meaning in light of this report.

Is a higher sperm count better? Not necessarily. Provided that the sperm are motile (capable of moving) and not malformed, it doesn't matter where your count ranks within the norm. After all, for a viable pregnancy all you need is one healthy sperm to fertilize one healthy, accessible egg. So 20 million per milliliter is perfectly acceptable in the scheme of reproductive abilities.

Are sperm counts declining around the world? Consensus among the medical community is no, despite a long-term regional study in Scandinavia that made a media splash in 1992 by reporting a big dropoff. The Danish researcher who made this claim has been tracking sperm counts since 1938. His observation: Modern environmental pollutants are wreaking havoc on sperm production. Other reports confirm sperm counts to be lower in third world countries. The Society for Male Reproduction and Urology (SMRU), a division of the American Society for Reproductive Medicine, is investigating this possible trend. Last word from the U.S. experts, published in May 1996, reports no decline in quality, volume, or percentage of normal sperm since 1972.

Can you build up sperm count? Yes, somewhat, by cutting back on alcoholic beverages and smoking and by trying vitamin E therapy. Avoiding restrictive underwear may help, and it is certainly worth the small investment in boxer shorts. Some studies show that increasing your caffeine intake may actually build up your sperm count. If you are diagnosed with a hormonal imbalance, the fertility drugs associated with IVF (Clomid, Pergonal, and hCG) may act as an antidote. But the best news for male factor infertility is that even if you produce only one single sperm, or none at all, the new technology may be able to work for you.

See: ICSI (intracytoplasmic sperm injection)

26. MOTILITY AND MORPHOLOGY: *How do the measures of speed and shape for sperm influence fertility? What does the swim up test prove?*

The urologist will check that your sperm can move effectively and that it looks normal. Motility measures the sperm's ability to travel through a woman's reproductive tract in order to meet her egg. Speed is the issue here. At least half of the sample should prove motile— i.e., 30 million in a count of 60 million per milliliter. Morphology—"shape" in lay terms—is analyzed for abnormalities that may be impeding its ability to fertilize. Basically the sperm should have a normal head and a single tail for optimal results. What does a healthy sperm look like? Typically it has the appearance of a balloon on a string with an oval head atop a long curly tail. (An abnormal sperm may have two heads, two tails, or a misshapen head.) Again, the norm is that half the sample should conform to the proper shape.

If motility is in question, the urologist will look into possible hormonal imbalances. Blood tests can measure how the thyroid and pituitary glands are functioning as well as levels of the secretion of sex hormones. The same fertility drugs that stimulate the female ovaries are used to regulate male hormones.

When both shape and count fall within the normal range, yet the sperm doesn't have the ability to fertilize an egg, the sperm may have a swimming problem. They may be clumping either because of infection or injury to the sperm ducts. Or antibodies present in the man's bloodstream may be negatively impacting sperm production.

In order to check whether movement is an issue, a sperm sample is inserted into columns of the medium called Percoll. Like Olympic swimmers, the sperm is then expected to make its way up to the finish line from the starting point. If debris is a problem, it will be sifted out through this process in order to create a potent sample of healthy sperm. For maximum penetration power, the final sample may be stored with other substances, such as test yolk buffer or follicle fluid skimmed off at the time of egg retrieval.

Penetration of the egg by the sperm is essential in the equation of making a baby. Standard tests measure this trait by watching how the sperm combines with either a hamster or human ovum. In the former scenario (the zona-free hamster egg penetration test) chemically treated hamster eggs are mixed with sperm in a lab dish. Since there is no possibility of ensuing embryos, the results are simply measured by how many eggs are successfully penetrated. Unfortunately, the margin of error is rather wide; normal results have been proved wrong, and some "failed" cases have been known to impregnate their partners at a later date. More accurate—and more rarely administered—is the hemi-zona test, using the eggs of cadavers or surgically removed human ovaries. (Human eggs are aspirated in order to prevent the development of embryos.) Once again the sperm are measured for the power of penetration into the human egg to determine if they can fertilize the egg without micromanipulation by an embryologist.

In the past, failing the hamster test meant moving on to donor sperm. These days the new ICSI procedure in concert with IVF may have an excellent prognosis.

27. SPERM WASHING (SPERM SEPARATION): *How does sperm washing improve quality? When is it indicated?*

Sperm washing is required prior to intrauterine insemination (IUI) or to enhance a sample and does not imply that natural sperm is unclean. What this process does is separate the active from the suboptimal sperm and the rest of the liquid ejaculate. You may hear reference to Percoll separation, which is the sperm-washing fluid of choice.

During sexual intercourse sperm enters the reproductive tract through the cervix. At that juncture the sperm's head cover (acrosome) reacts to the cervical mucus by releasing enzymes that prepare it to penetrate the egg. This preamble to fertilization is called capacitation.

With IUI capacitation must be artificially simulated. Since the fertility practitioner injects the chemically treated sperm directly into the uterus via a catheter, the cervix is bypassed altogether and can neither filter the semen nor initiate capacitation. Sperm washing removes those chemical substances in the semen (prostaglandins) that may induce painful uterine contractions. The laboratory technician combines the sample with a sterile fluid (Percoll) in a centrifuge to isolate the sperm from the fluids (seminal plasma). The heavier healthy sperm move to the bottom and are sifted out.

Washed sperm is stored in a small vial of medium at body temperature (37 degrees Celsius) until the insemination appointment. The Percoll is washed away prior to insemination. If the sperm is left in the solution for 24 hours, capacitation will begin. Since washing extracts the healthy sperm, it should be in Olympic form, which may enhance fertilization if all the other variables are in place.

28. VARICOCELES (VARICOSE VEINS IN THE GROIN): Why do some men develop varicoceles? Can they be cured?

Just as varicose veins can develop in legs, so they may appear in the scrotum. This may be a birth defect associated with your mother's use of DES, or it may be the luck of the draw. Some may be obvious; others are detected during physical exams or with ultrasound. High levels of abnormally shaped sperm or low motility in a semen analysis usually lead to this diagnosis.

Enlarged veins (varicoceles) raise the temperature

around the testes and reduce sperm production. Depending on sperm count, if this condition is caught in the early stage, the urologist may choose to tie off the veins using X-ray visualization in order to improve semen quality. When the sperm count is very low, the urologist will examine other factors (FSH level, obstruction of the vas deferens or epididymis).

Keeping sperm at the right temperature is a key consideration in maximizing their potency. Ideally the scrotum should be slightly cooler than the body temperature in order to keep up the production of healthy sperm. Varicosed veins in the testicles (varicoceles) may turn the internal thermostat up in the scrotum by preventing good blood circulation. For men in fertility treatment, varicoceles follow sexually transmitted disease as a leading diagnosis.

If your urologist considers you a good candidate, semen quality may improve following a varicocelectomy. This ambulatory procedure entails closing off the affected site through X-ray visualization. To gain access to the area, incisions are made above the groin. Recovery is comparable to hernia repair surgery. How successful is a varicocelectomy in reestablishing fertility? Not very, according to eminent specialists such as Robert Winston, M.D., director of Britain's largest IVF program at Hammersmith Hospital. Lord Winston blames poor training for the ineffectiveness of this microsurgery. Statistics show one in five untreated cases will succeed in impregnating his partner, exactly comparable to the odds following surgery. But whether or not you opt for surgery, the varicocele must be followed during annual physicals to ensure that it hasn't changed size and compromised sperm production any further.

The trend today for the man with suboptimal sperm is to go straight for IVF (via ICSI) or donor insemination rather than to treat the individual problem. The introduction and good results of ICSI, which works through the injection of sperm into the egg, have rendered other technologies obsolete.

29. TESTICULAR BIOPSY (LAB ANALYSIS): When is a testicular biopsy called for?

If your sperm count is near zero, your diagnosis may be oligozoospermia or azoospermia: low or no sperm production. A biopsy can determine the underlying reason, which may be due to either structural or hormonal causes. About 5% of male factor is the result of the latter. In the case of a low sperm count yet a normal FSH, the doctor may find structural blockage. Simple microsurgery may be able to undo the obstruction and cure the problem. Under local or general anesthesia, the urologist will remove a small sample of the tissue from the testicles for analysis in the lab.

If infection is detected, antibiotic therapy may offer a quick and simple cure. Any prior history of venereal disease or tuberculosis should be included in your health profile to help your doctor determine why you are not producing sperm.

See: Male factor—no sperm

30. MALE HORMONE ISSUES: How are male hormone imbalances corrected?

The key hormones in the universe of reproduction for both sexes are follicle-stimulating hormone (FSH) and luteinizing hormone (LH). They are controlled jointly from the brain by the pituitary gland and the hypothalamus. A proper chain of events in men stimulates sperm manufacture: The LH triggers production of the male hormone (testosterone) within the testes, while the FSH nurtures the immature sperm cells to develop fully. Disorders of the thyroid or prolactin hormones may take a toll on sperm production as well.

The same medicine cabinet of fertility drugs routinely used for women applies here as well. If your andrologist finds that pituitary function is at the root of the problem, a prescription of low-dose Clomid either daily or every other day may stimulate FSH and LH production. Where the deficiency is severe, the protocol may escalate to Pergonal and Metrodin three times a week for up to six months. Parlodel is indicated to correct hypothyroidism, while hCG injections twice a week should boost testosterone. Side effects from these prescriptions include weight gain and moodiness that may manifest itself as a short fuse.

Are these medications effective? It's difficult to discern, and studies are inconclusive. With sperm levels varying drastically from sample to sample, experts are having trouble distinguishing between natural variation and improvement caused by treatment. For men with severe problems, ICSI may be the more effective treatment.

31. PERFORMANCE ANXIETY: *How can we overcome performance anxiety? With the calendar staring us in the face each month, my husband is having trouble keeping an erection.*

Spontaneity is the first casualty of fertility treatment. Nothing puts a crimp in your sex life like following the calendar, charting your sexual activity, and being required to perform on appointed days. Sometimes just the prospect of providing a sample for the lab may create a level of stress that makes masturbation impossible for some men. A loss of self-esteem and resulting guilt feelings about being "responsible" for the fertility problem can complicate matters further.

If you are undergoing insemination or IVF and are worried about getting a sample in time for the procedure, it may be advisable to freeze sperm in advance as insurance. Although it is not the preferred method, your doctor can provide a special condom that collects the specimen during intercourse.

Keep in mind that the love you share with your partner led you into treatment in the first place. Address these conflicted feelings together or with your specialist. Sometimes short-term psychological counseling may help you through a difficult time on your journey to building a family.

32. MALE FACTOR—NO SPERM (AZOOSPERMIA): Is it true that a new technique is being used in conjunction with IVF that can capture the few good sperm to create a viable pregnancy? My husband's sperm production has been analyzed as next to nothing.

Yes, an amazing recent development has made pregnancy possible despite low or nonexistent sperm counts. Introduced in Belgium in 1993, this option has quickly gained acceptance in the United States. When used together with IVF, this technique, popularly known as ICSI (intracytoplasmic sperm injection, pronounced *ick-see*), reports a fertilization rate of nearly 80%. The take-home-baby rate compares with standard IVF without ICSI, depending upon your age. If you have a male factor problem (no sperm, abnormal shape, not motile), ICSI offers tremendous hope.

All the embryologist needs to create a viable embryo with this technique is a single sperm per egg. Rather than allow sperm and egg to fertilize spontaneously in the petri dish, with ICSI the sperm is injected directly into the egg with a thin glass needle. To date ICSI has been proved to work for men with a variety of severe quality issues from low counts (below one million) to azoospermia, in which the ejaculate contains no sperm at all. The technique has gained such support in the medical community that it promises to become part of the standard IVF procedure in the future. Right now, however, it is not yet widely available in every ART facility because it requires specialized equipment.

Another new development in the field is known as percutaneous epididymal sperm aspiration (PESA) plus ICSI. This procedure is recommended for men with no sperm caused by a vasectomy or an absent vas deferens. Under local sedation, semen is aspirated from the epididymis with a series of punctures. In conjunction with ICSI and ovarian stimulation in the woman, successful pregnancies have been achieved this way in seven of 13 patients in a recent case study. Four of these pregnancies were multiples (three sets of twins and one set of triplets).

An ice pack applied to the scrotal area should alleviate postoperative discomfort. Studies are showing better results with this technique than with surgical vasectomy reversal. Does low sperm quality translate into an increase in birth defects for babies born of this technique? Not according to current research. To monitor congenital defects in ICSI embryos, some clinics recommend karyotyping of the male partner. Although it may be too soon to draw definitive conclusions, studies as recent as 1996 report birth defects in about 3% of babies born through IVF with or without ICSI, comparable to the national average.

FEMALE FACTORS

33. OVULATION: *How can I track ovulation? How many eggs do I produce monthly? Is it possible for the ovaries to ovulate but not release an egg? I have been diagnosed with luteinized unruptured follicle (LUF) syndrome.*

You are born with two ovaries that contain a wealth of eggs. The average woman starts her reproductive life with a store of about 300,000 eggs. At the onset of menstruation, around the age of 13, the ovaries begin to expel one mature egg per month. If you assume that you will be ovulating for another 40 years, your body's natural production of mature eggs could reach a total of 500. For every mature egg, your body also expels another 500 or so small ones per cycle, which are reabsorbed by the body. Although in theory you will not deplete your supply until menopause, you may run out of viable eggs capable of being fertilized by the time you reach your early forties.

The monthly chain of events begins when the cells around a single egg develop to create a fluid-filled sac (Graafian follicle). When the follicle reaches a full-grown size of about 20 millimeters, the fimbriae sweep the egg out of the sac and into the fallopian tubes, and ovulation takes place. Once empty, the follicle (corpus luteum) collapses and assumes a yellow hue. Each month one of your two ovaries releases many follicles, one of which will develop into an egg (ovum). The egg develops in the two weeks following your last period. When the egg is penetrated by a sperm, the fertilized egg embeds itself into the endometrium, which nourishes the growing embryo. Sometimes two eggs are released or one splits into two. If this is the case and fertilization occurs, you will have twins. Unless conception takes place, though, the egg will be discarded along with the lining of your uterus about two weeks later when your next period begins.

Ovulation relies on the production of three groups of hormones: estrogens, androgens, and progesterone. Ensuring the timely development and release of the follicle in this delicate recipe are two key secretions: follicle-stimulating hormone (FSH) and luteinizing hormone (LH), which are released by the pituitary gland. A deficiency of any of these hormones may result in ovulation factor infertility. In the case of LUF syndrome, the ovaries take egg development only up to the point before release so that fertilization can't take place.

The average menstrual cycle is 28 days, although the normal range spans from 25 to 32 days. Ovulation occurs 14 days before the next period begins. If we call the first day of bleeding Day 1, your body will begin exhibiting signals that ovulation is imminent on or about Day 13 of the 28-day cycle. At this time you will notice increased discharge from the vagina. As the egg is growing in the ovary, your body is producing higher levels of the female hormone called estradiol. In turn this hormone secretes a clear mucus that you will notice upon wiping the vaginal area. At first the mucus is sticky and thick. Once it assumes the look of an egg white, more see-through and elastic, ovulation is imminent. After the egg is released, the amount of mucus diminishes again.

If you don't have any reservations about examining the mucus yourself, you may want to try the "Billings Method." It requires you to hold a sample of the mucus between your thumb and forefinger. If you don't notice any stretch, you know you are in the early part of your cycle. Your cervix is not yet open, and the egg is in the early stage of development. Eventually the mucus should thin out, and you will be able to extend the fingers up to three inches without breaking it. That is the signal that ovulation is due to occur in the next 36 to 72 hours.

For the more scientific soul, pharmaceutical companies have designed ovulation kits. These neat boxes are sold in drugstores for from about $15 (First Response) to more than $65* (OvuQUICK). My gynecologist recommended the Q-test ($25). By measuring the amount of LH in the urine, these kits pinpoint ovulation. Levels of LH rise as the egg matures and drop off after it is released. Is it possible to get your period regularly without releasing an egg? Yes, in some cases, such as if you have polycystic ovaries.

For women who enjoy predictable and regular cycles, the kit system works nicely. For example, if you have a 28-day cycle, you begin to test your urine on Day 11. Perform the test at the same time each morning in order to have the most concentrated sample. For best results, don't drink anything for one hour beforehand since liquids may dilute the LH level. (You may refrigerate the sample and test later in the day, if time is scarce.) Within a couple of days you'll notice a shift in response. For women with irregular cycles, you may have to test your urine for up to 10 days in order to capture the day of ovulation.

See: Polycystic ovarian syndrome

34. OVULATION/OVARIAN RESERVE SCREENING (CLOMID CHALLENGE TEST): Can my ovaries "run dry"? Is there a way to find out?

The question is not whether your ovaries are running out of eggs so much as whether they're running low on viable ones. A screening test can determine if a woman is approaching menopause by measuring the hormone levels in her blood on Day 3 of her menstrual cycle. Results before and after ovarian stimulation will give your practitioner a more accurate picture of your ovarian function. As long as your follicle-stimulating hormone (FSH) level is less than 15 mIU/ml and your estradiol (estrogen) is under 75 pg/ml, you're considered fertile. Once the doctor knows that your ovaries are productive, you will be advised on the best course of action for you.

That you have a monthly period is no guarantee you are either ovulating or fertile. In fact, over the course of six years leading up to menopause, your infertility index shoots way up. For example, if menopause is going to occur at age 51, the average in the United States, your body is beginning to shut down its production of female hormones at age 44. Not even the miracles of ART can work against the forces of nature. IVF success rates for women age 43 or over are negligible when using their own eggs. For women between 40 and 42, an estimated one in 10 will produce her own biological baby through IVF. With GIFT, success is better at about one in six women. What's more upsetting, the risk of miscarriages is elevated for this age group.

Is there a way to bank eggs when you're young, just

as men are able to bank their sperm? Not as of this writing. Eggs are too fragile to undergo freezing and thawing with any measure of success. Embryos, however, are more resilient and are successfully surviving the cryopreservation process. But making embryos for future use is still neither feasible nor economical.

Are women reaching menopause earlier? No trend has been recognized officially, and population studies demonstrate no change in the onset age of menopause over the last 100 years. Perhaps the diagnosis of premature ovarian failure is simply symptomatic of this generation of career women. In the past women with this syndrome either had babies young or couldn't pursue pregnancy since the technology didn't exist. Our good fortune is that technology is catching up with our personal goals.

See: Day 3 (below)

35. DAY 3 BLOODWORK: *What do the hormone levels on Day 3 reveal about my fertility?*

Each cycle begins on the first day of your period, referred to as Day 1, which introduces the follicular phase. Hormones within the ovary are collaborating to produce a mature follicle that will release an egg (ovum) around Day 14. On Day 3 blood is drawn to measure the level of two female hormones, follicle-stimulating hormone (FSH) and estradiol (estrogen). A third hormone, inhibin B, has recently been shown to be a reliable prognostic tool in a study at Brown University's School of Medicine.

Until your body experiences the surge of luteinizing hormone (LH) on the day before ovulation, the numbers will be expected to rise as the dominant follicle develops within the ovary. For example, Day 3 may show an FSH under 13 (mIU/ml) and an LH under 7.

Ideally, at Day 13 both levels will have exceeded 15 mIU/ml, and your estradiol should pass 100 pg/ml. Meanwhile, for best results the inhibin B level should exceed 45 pg/ml. An overall increase indicates that an egg has developed within the dominant follicle to its full size (about an inch). By following the measure of your hormone levels, your doctor can assess ovarian function in order to determine the appropriate dosage of fertility drugs and how well your body will respond to them.

As you approach menopause (climacteric, in the clinical term), ovarian function begins to shut down. For the average woman this process begins about six years prior to her last period, when she reaches her 44th birthday. One of the symptoms of this decline is elevated FSH on Day 3. This shift indicates that the production of a dominant follicle is being discontinued. Since FSH levels fluctuate from month to month, however, your doctor should review more than one cycle before drawing any conclusions. Keep in mind too that some 43-year-old women may respond like women 10 years their junior. That makes generalizations based on age difficult.

With the onset of menopause, your ovaries will not respond sufficiently no matter how large a dose of fertility drugs is administered. While you will produce one or two eggs under normal circumstances, fertility medication boosts results to dozens per cycle in a fertile woman. Where do the extra eggs come from? Normally the ovary produces a single mature egg while expelling the immature ones, which are absorbed back into the body. Fertility drugs work to "rescue" and cultivate these immature eggs into fully developed, viable ones in order to increase the potential number of embryos. Since the principle behind ART procedures is to enhance the odds of implantation of a single embryo by transferring many, the more healthy embryos you have, the higher degree of success you may achieve.

36. HYSTEROSALPINGOGRAM (HSG): What will the hysterosalpingogram show about my fallopian tubes? Why do I have to sign a release? How do I know if I'm allergic to the dye? . . . HYSTEROSCOPY: When do I need a hysteroscopy?

Most workups begin with this hard-to-pronounce test, which is scheduled in the second week of your cycle. In order to get pregnant, you need proof that your fallopian tubes are up to performing their job, which is to guide the unfertilized egg into the uterus, and that your uterus is properly shaped to carry a full-term baby. Blockage caused by scar tissue resulting from endometriosis or a past infection may be preventing the egg from meeting a sperm. To determine if the tubes are open and functioning, your doctor will arrange for a hysterosalpingogram (HSG), an X ray of the tubes and uterus. Results from the HSG will indicate whether your diagnosis is due to a uterine or tubal factor.

Is this procedure uncomfortable? Yes, it is. But thankfully it is over in about 40 minutes. (A prophylactic tab of ibuprofen or a mild tranquilizer taken prior to the test may help alleviate anxiety and discomfort.) In order to protect the uterus from bacteria that may enter it during the test, you will need to be on antibiotic therapy. As with any X ray, you are exposed to radiation. In this case the dose is minimal—between one and two rads.

First, you must remove your clothes and put on a hospital gown. After you are settled on an examining table, a special type of speculum (tenaculum) is inserted into the vagina to hold the cervix in place. An iodine-based (standard contrast) solution is injected directly through the cervix into the uterus and, it is hoped, into the fallopian tubes. For women who are allergic to shellfish or are concerned about potential allergies, an equivalent water-based substitute is used. As you lie on a large table, the X ray stares down at you from the ceiling. You'll experience a pinch when the needle penetrates the cervix.

As the solution fills the area, a technician takes a series of X rays of the left and right hips (about 15 or 20 minutes per hip). Ideally the dye, which registers as a shadow, flows through the tubes and spills freely into the uterus. Once the films are developed, tubal function and the outline of the organs can be assessed. The diameter of the cervix will be checked to rule out the possibility of an incompetent cervix. Obvious blockages, fibroid tumors, or structural abnormalities will be revealed immediately.

Since the solution leaks out afterward, you must wear a sanitary pad for the rest of the day. You may experience residual cramping that can be preempted with your chosen over-the-counter medication. Some clinics suggest that you arrange to have someone take you home, for you may be in some discomfort. The degree of discomfort depends on the condition of your tubes as well as your personal tolerance level. The first time I arranged for an HSG during a lunch hour, which worked well for me. However, the nurses were alarmed and insisted that I contact my husband and leave word that I might need to be picked up. I went ahead with the test and returned to my office afterward. A tab of ibuprofen counteracted the residual discomfort. My gynecologist (not a reproductive endocrinologist) read the films on the spot and told me my tubes were fine.

More encouraging than the good results was the

news that this test may have therapeutic benefits. Apparently the dye can temporarily flush aside scar tissue. Some doctors estimate that pregnancy rates may improve by as much as 50% after an HSG. But the window of opportunity is brief because the tissue tends to return. If you haven't conceived by the cycle following the test, you may safely assume that your tubes have reclosed. The same principle may apply to laser surgery for blocked tubes; scar tissue grows back by the next cycle. Fertility specialists no longer recommend repair surgery for severely blocked or swollen tubes since as a rule IVF shows better results for tubal factor. While the emotional desire to conceive naturally may always remain in the back of your mind, you've got to work with your body to make your wish a reality.

In my case, another 24 cycles with no pregnancy elapsed before my RE had me redo the test on a hunch. (Again I went unescorted.) Diagnosis: tubal factor caused by PID. Although I had been married a decade by that point and had never had a pelvic infection in my life, at least to my knowledge, it was a relief to pinpoint a reason I wasn't conceiving.

While an HSG is a standard part of the workup, there are some considerations you must address. First, you will be asked to sign a waiver. This piece of paper will bring to your attention the fact that when a foreign substance containing a nonsoluble dye enters your reproductive tract, you risk infection. In an estimated 2% of cases the dye may turn a dormant infection into an active case of pelvic inflammatory disease that will create serious obstruction. For patients with histories of known PID it may be advisable to forgo this test and move on to a laparoscopy or hysteroscopy in order to contain any possible risk of a flare-up.

Secondly, doctors acknowledge that the HSG is not

entirely foolproof. In fact, there is a slim chance of a faulty reading, which may send you back for a retest. How can an X ray be wrong? Shadows may fall in such a way as to cloud results, or scar tissue may not show up clearly. As a result, the initial diagnosis may not be accurate. What's more, the HSG doesn't offer a full picture of the connection between the fallopian tubes and the ovaries; scar tissue around the ovaries may be blocking the egg's progress into the reproductive tract despite the proper functioning of tubes and uterus. If you are scheduled for a laparoscopy (an ambulatory procedure that assesses your reproductive organs), you may inquire whether you can skip the HSG.

As for hysteroscopy, it is primarily indicated when uterine factor is the expected diagnosis. Symptoms that may precede the procedure include a history of fibroid tumors, pelvic inflammatory disease, or irregular bleeding. This microsurgical technique, indicated most often where peritoneal factor is suspected, may be performed in the doctor's office under local anesthesia or in the operating room under general anesthesia. After 60 minutes or more in the recovery room, you will be released.

In this procedure, which takes about half an hour, a lighted scope is inserted into the vagina, then through the dilated cervix into the lower end of the uterus. By injecting carbon dioxide into the area, the doctor can examine the internal structure of the womb through the scope. Many small growths (fibroids, polyps, or post-surgical scars from Asherman's syndrome) can be removed at this time via the hysteroscope. A new technique called sonohysteroscopy is being introduced as an initial screening tool in identifying polyps and similar growths. When a saline solution is infused into the uterus, the endometrial cavity can be examined with a simple sonogram.

Congenital anomalies such as a septate (split) uterus can be corrected with laser or the use of surgical scissors through this method as well. The side effects are the same as with the HSG—namely, cramping and staining. Scar tissue resulting from Asherman's syndrome may be removed in order to restore endometrial function. If there has been any corrective action, you may expect some residual bleeding for one or two days. Since this is a relatively new technology, it's in your best interest to recruit a doctor with experience in this delicate procedure.

37. ENDOMETRIAL BIOPSY: What does an endometrial biopsy involve? I've heard it's painful.

In this test the doctor takes a sample of your endometrium (uterine lining) just prior to your period and sends it to the laboratory for analysis. During this part of the cycle the endometrium should be rich in estrogen and progesterone in order to nurture the fertilized egg. If the lining is not primed to do its job, it could undermine your attempts to get pregnant.

The sample is removed with a small curette or suction device that is threaded through the cervix. This procedure is generally performed during an office visit without the benefit of any anesthesia. Advil or Valium may help you through this 60-second endurance test. I've heard some degree of discomfort is involved, first when the instrument enters the cervix and later when the sample is taken. Subsequent cramping may occur, and you can expect some spotting.

Biopsy results help the doctor confirm what blood and urine tests may be indicating: that hormone levels (specifically progesterone) are below normal levels during the seven days following ovulation (the luteal phase). The conclusion is based on a report by the pathology lab after it has examined the cells of the uterine lining in light of the date of ovulation. If you're diagnosed with a luteal phase deficiency (LPD), you will move on to hormone therapy. Perhaps a history of early miscarriage has preceded this diagnosis. What other factors may require this test? Any problem that may be compromising embryo implantation, including unexplained infertility. But unless one of these factors is present, this test is no longer a mandatory part of the standard workup.

See: Blood test, Progesterone

38. LAPAROSCOPY: When is a laparoscopy called for? Does it mean entering the operating room? Is it uncomfortable? Are there any nonsurgical alternatives? What is an augmented laparoscopy?

Although many inferences about your case can be made on the basis of other workup tests, a laparoscopy allows the doctor to diagnose definitively tubal or peritoneal factors by giving him or her a bird's-eye view into your pelvis. As of the mid-1990s, however, this procedure is no longer considered a mandatory part of the workup but rather an alternative to IVF. If your practitioner can surmise tubal factor based on results of the balance of the workup, IVF may be recommended over laparoscopy.

The laparoscope, a thin viewing instrument with a telescopic lens, is inserted through or just below your belly button via a small incision. Carbon dioxide is pumped into the abdomen to allow for better viewing. Through the scope the microsurgeon looks for adhesions or scar tissue on the peritoneum (pelvic lining), ovaries, or tubes that he or she may be able to remove during this procedure. Usually, by the time you reach this stage, your doctor will have a hunch about what is going on inside on the basis of the results of the other tests.

Since an exploratory or diagnostic laparoscopy is potentially the most extensive part of your workup, it takes place in the hospital under general anesthesia with all the anxieties and protocol that any operation entails. The night before the procedure you will be asked not to eat or drink anything after midnight. At the hospital you check your belongings in a locker and change into a hospital gown. (Leave jewelry at home for safekeeping since you will be asked to remove it.) Your husband or companion may accompany you to the waiting room.

During the procedure, which takes half an hour or so, about four liters of carbon dioxide gas will be pumped into a small incision in your abdomen to allow for greater visibility into the area. In the recovery room you may feel pain in the shoulder area as the gas moves through your bloodstream. Typical reactions to anesthesia include nausea and teariness. Or if you're like me, you may lie prone for four and a half hours until the general anesthesia has completely worn off.

Since your stomach will be slightly distended from the gas, it's best to wear loose-fitting pants. Except for residual light-headedness from the anesthesia, recovery usually does not extend beyond 24 hours. The stitches in your belly button will dissolve within the week, and the scar will be unnoticeable.

An augmented laparoscopy entails more than a simple exam of the area. If there is reason to believe that your tubes are blocked, for example, your doctor may recommend combining a GIFT procedure with the laparoscopy. After checking the area and removing any small growths, the doctor would then transfer the embryo(s) through the laparoscope.

39. ULTRASOUND: How does sonography work? How can it measure follicular development? Does it hurt?

To ensure that your ovaries are indeed producing mature eggs at least 14 mm in diameter, your fertility practice should have an on-site transvaginal ultrasound device with a full-time technician. Like X rays, ultrasound allows the doctor to see what's going on inside your body. Unlike X rays, no known dangerous side effects are associated with this test; sonography operates on the principle of sound waves rather than radiation. This technology has been around for more than 20 years and has been shown to be a safe mode of examination. In fact, it's considered so safe that it is used throughout the course of pregnancy to monitor the fetus.

Once you are on a fertility drug protocol, your follicular development will be closely monitored via ultrasound, and your blood will be drawn to keep tabs on hormone levels. Depending upon how your body responds to the medication, somewhere around Day 14 you may be scheduled for an egg retrieval.

The ultrasound transducer (which resembles a hard plastic tampon) "looks" inside the uterine cavity and "reads" high-frequency sound waves traveling through the area. These sonogram images appear on a TV monitor almost like a radar to help the practitioner identify what's going on in the uterine cavity. After the LH surge, the collapsed follicle should be visible, and that means the egg is on its way. Measurements on the uterine lining should begin to increase as it thickens in preparation for receiving the fertilized egg. No physical discomfort is associated with these internal snapshots—after you get over any initial embarrassment.

You may follow your progress on the screen, where

you can clearly see your ovaries and, one hopes, the growing follicles. Watching the eggs ripen for harvest can be an encouraging experience. As the transducer focuses on each individual follicle, the technician takes the measurements in millimeters. By analyzing the size of the follicles together with the elevation of estradiol in the blood, your doctor can make a determination about the timing of the hCG shot that ultimately triggers ovulation.

BOTH OF YOU:
CERVICAL FACTOR

40. POSTCOITAL TEST: *What will the postcoital test (PCT or Huhner) test prove?*

Just when you thought you could stop performing by the calendar and leave everything to medical science, your doctor will ask you to have sex at home one more time. This part of the workup should precede ovulation and coincide with the LH surge when mucus is most receptive to sperm. (At another point in the cycle, readings may not be accurate.) Within two hours or so after, the doctor will swab a sample from your vagina and send it to the laboratory for analysis. Results will reveal whether sperm can swim freely and survive in the environment. At the same time bacterial screening will uncover possible infections. If the sperm appear immotile, the diagnosis is cervical factor.

Cervical factor accounts for about one in 20 fertility problems. The related diagnosis includes the (lack of) quantity or quality of the mucus or the presence of antibodies. As the passageway between the vagina and the uterus, the cervix must welcome sperm into the reproductive tract. During the cycle the cervical canal changes shape. When ovulation occurs, the cervix invites sperm in by shifting forward, opening the canal, and secreting more mucus. A problem with cervical mucus accounts for about 5% of fertility problems.

What causes the quality of mucus to drop? First, check that the PCT was performed at the correct time of month. Other explanations include exposure to DES, a cone biopsy, or other treatment for cervical cancer. (Following a bad Pap smear, sometimes a cone biopsy is indicated to remove precancerous tissue.)

Treatment of cervical factor depends on the problem. If antibodies are lurking in the mucus, intrauterine insemination (IUI) may do the trick. Bacterial problems can be cured with antibiotics. For improved quality, your RE may prescribe hormone therapy.

41. ASSISTED REPRODUCTIVE TECHNOLOGY: When do we move on to ART? What if we don't feel ready?

The decision on whether to continue with ART is wholly up to you and your partner. Although our generation is the first to have the option of using reproductive technology, it is a voluntary choice based on financial and emotional limits. While your doctor can advise you on the medical course appropriate to you, you have to be receptive to what treatment entails. Even 15 or 20 years ago a 35-year-old woman with blocked tubes, for example, would have been told that she had no chance of bearing children. Now she could end up having twins through in vitro if she elects to go that route.

To help you make an educated decision, you may wish to consult the "Guidelines for the Provision of Infertility Services," available from the American Society for Reproductive Medicine. By dividing care into three levels, you can see where you fall in the spectrum of treatment and determine which way you're headed.

Criteria that distinguish the levels include how long you've been trying, your age, past treatment, and any health risks. Level III represents the big guns, assisted reproductive technology.

Bear in mind, however, that ultimately nature may make this decision for you. A certain amount of ambivalence about changing your status to family after prolonged coupledom is to be expected. But biologically the window of opportunity is already half shut by the time you hit 40. Hormone tests can indicate whether your body is still producing good-quality gametes (sperm and eggs). But no tests guarantee how good-quality gametes will combine or whether they will produce healthy embryos to create full-term pregnancies. Emotionally and career-wise, timing may be a capricious factor. The world watched as television personalities Connie Chung and Maury Povich ultimately turned to adoption after sharing the fact of failing in vitro treatment when Chung was past 40.

Sometimes a diagnosis may put undue pressure on the member of the couple who has the fertility problem to pursue treatment. Feelings of guilt, resentment, confusion, or depression may arise in reaction. In cases of unexplained infertility, couples have confided that they were relieved that neither was "to blame." Keeping the lines of communication open between the two of you during this time will help you cope with this unexpected glitch in your life plan.

PART III

CAUSES

QUESTIONS ABOUT UNDERLYING REASONS FOR INFERTILITY

42. ADHESIONS: *What do the protrusions on the uterine wall that my doctor noted in a routine physical mean about my ability to conceive?*

Adhesions act like glue in the pelvis by connecting distant organs of the cavity and distorting their placement. Under normal circumstances, your internal organs are held in place by a membrane (peritoneum) that coats the abdominal wall. Once bacteria or trauma disturb the membrane, the mending process may result in the development of adhesions. Suddenly an ovary is stuck to the intestine, a tube is stuck to an ovary, or any number of other combinations may occur. Only by performing a laparoscopy will your RE be able to measure how extensive the adhesions may be.

Adhesions are bands of fibrous scar tissue that bind the pelvic organs together, and they develop from one of three causes: PID, pelvic surgery, or endometriosis. Insidiously an infection may have created a web of problems through PID that you are just learning about. Or you may recall an acute abdominal infection (appendicitis or peritonitis) or corrective surgery on an ovarian cyst. Unintentional damage to the peritoneum may take its toll on fertility.

Or adhesions may be symptomatic of a chronic condition caused by the appearance of polyps (benign lesions) in the endometrium. For example, endometrial glands may grow inside the uterine wall, and that could result in an enlarged uterus and bleeding. Or it could interfere with proper embryo implantation. Women over 40 are more susceptible to this development. If caught in time, this condition—adenomyosis—may respond to a prescription for estradiol valerate, a form of female hormone. In severe cases, in which pain becomes an issue, hysterectomy may be recommended.

Other abnormal growths in the uterine wall include fibroid tumors (myoma) and endometrioma. While the word *tumors* may evoke frightening images, in fact, fibroids are generally harmless growths that seldom compromise fertility. Surgical removal is indicated only if there is a sudden enlargement or if they create chronic pain. You will require further testing to get to the root of your real diagnosis. As for endometriosis, a new drug on the market has made big inroads in controlling the development of adhesions in the pelvis.

For adhesions caused by PID (pelvic inflammatory disease), two options are open to you: repair surgery or IVF. Naturally you will want to explore the possibility of repair first. If the adhesions are blocking your tubes, your doctor will discuss the prognosis of tuboplasty. Your chances of recovering tubal function are better if the blockage exists closer to the uterus rather than at the fimbriated end. Since scar tissue tends to recur quickly despite the surgeon's best efforts, however, the success of any repair surgery will be contingent upon the extent of the problem, your age, and the skill of your surgeon. In some cases a protocol of steroids, antibiotics, and tranquilizers following surgery may prevent adhesions from re-forming.

Unless you are under 35 or have a mild case, chances

are the specialist will recommend going directly for IVF. Since the peritoneum is so delicate, any surgery—even the repair—may cause new adhesions to form. Especially if the uterine lining (endometrium) is compromised in its function, fertility drug therapy in concert with IVF may have better results. Your eggs can then be fertilized outside the body, and the frozen embryos may be replaced in your uterus during a future cycle when your endometrium is in its natural state. In the event that your endometrium cannot support a pregnancy, you may even consider the use of a gestational host.

See: Endometriosis, Fibroids

43. AGE-RELATED FACTORS: Part a) Aged 40, and over (perimenopause): How significant is age to my ability to have a baby in the near future? I am a 40-year-old newlywed. My mother gave birth to me when she was over 40, and I read about celebrities like Kathie Lee Gifford and Jane Seymour who have had babies after 40 in recent times. I feel young and vibrant and have twice the energy I did 10 years ago. Yet I hear doctors won't treat women over 40.

Age has become the most critical factor in the business of making babies, according to expert consensus. The worst advice anyone can give you is to put career building ahead of starting a family, according to Dr. Jamie Grifo, director of reproductive endocrinology at the NYU Medical Center, who is expressing current medical wisdom. Unfortunately, millions of working people over 30 have reached this conclusion through experience and are seeking fertility treatment today. Don't assume that couples "of a certain age" (especially celebrities) got pregnant the old-fashioned way: Family planning nowadays often entails enlisting medical intervention.

A woman's egg begins to show signs of genetic deterioration after age 35, with the rate of abnormal chromosomes increasing sharply after age 40. As a result, the incidence of miscarriage rises with age as the body rejects these unsound embryos. The rate of miscarriage more than triples from 10% to nearly 34% between the time you're in your late twenties and your early forties. This is an indication that there are genetic defects in the embryos that prevent full-term development.

But what can you do if you meet the man of your dreams after age 35? If you haven't conceived after six months of unprotected intercourse, then the most effective course of action is to consult a specialist to find out why. What if the diagnosis is age-related and you choose to continue treatment? Learn about the options open to you and your husband. In the arena of assisted reproductive technology (ART) after age 40 donor eggs may be your best bet.

As you weigh the alternatives, the notion of carrying a pregnancy that is not biologically yours will not match the scenario that you had in mind. Yet the donor egg was bound to be the next logical step to follow sperm banks, which have been around for years. Rates of take-home babies with this procedure hover at 60% for most programs. Just as with adoption, the notion of raising a nonbiological child is an emotional issue to be addressed together with your partner or with a professional. The donor may be a relative or a stranger, depending on availability and which you are more comfortable choosing. An informal survey on my part seems to indicate that most women prefer anonymous donors.

Many women are devastated when their doctors give them the odds of conceiving with their own eggs. "My chances are one in 1,000 according to my doctor," a

42-year-old woman whispered to me in complete defeat. Recognize that it is the doctor's responsibility to give you the cold facts so that you can make an informed decision. Bring your partner to the doctor's office so that both of you hear the information at the same time and can support each other.

Part b) Aged 35 and under: Does infertility afflict young, healthy couples? My husband and I are both 28, and haven't used contraception since we married two years ago. We were planning to have a big family, yet so far we haven't conceived. Should I be concerned?

Yes, unfortunately, factors that cause infertility may appear in couples throughout the reproductive spectrum. High energy and good health are not a guarantee that all systems inside are go. Age does not discriminate on issues of sperm quality, ovulation, or tubal disorders. Where there is a history of miscarriage, young couples may be struggling with the immunological syndromes (antibodies) just being identified by the medical community.

Despite the urgency you may feel to start your family right now, in terms of treatment you have one advantage that money can't buy: time. Depending upon your diagnosis, you may have to rework your personal agenda somewhat and broaden your medical knowledge of the reproductive system. But with age 35 as the turning point for quality of genetic material the window of opportunity is wide open—provided that you enlist professional help soon. Enrolling in an accredited program and getting a diagnosis is the first step on the road to success.

44. ANATOMICAL ANOMALIES (CONGENITAL DEFECTS): *Since I was born with one fallopian tube (or one ovary, or a split uterus), where do I start medical treatment for a birth defect of my reproductive system?*

For the average fertility patient the prospect of medical intervention may come as a complete shock. The woman born with a Müllerian anomaly (an abnormal uterus), however, may have already come to terms with the role that treatment could play in her effort toward building a family. Any of three deviations (anomalies) from the normal appearance of the female organs (the Müllerian duct system) may arise: disorders of descent, disorders of fusion, and dysgenesis. Repair surgery with or without ART may lead to success for the first two anomalies. For women with dysgenesis (absent uterus and cervix), ART has devised the option of combining IVF with a host uterus (gestational carrier).

A disorder of descent refers to the way your fallopian tubes developed within Week 14 in the womb. In the normal configuration the tubes fuse and connect to the uterine cavity in a triangular shape. If they don't fuse properly at the point of entry to the vagina, symptoms may arise in childbearing years. Typically, an imperforate hymen may appear and act as a trap for menstrual blood. Eventually the trapped blood may develop into a pelvic cyst. This membrane can be surgically removed, and if no other fertility factors exist, you're in luck. As long as you are ovulating regularly, you may be able to conceive naturally.

A disorder of fusion, which also takes place early in fetal development, presents as a distortion in the uterine shape. Normally the shape resembles the appearance of a ram's head with the tubes representing the horns. The abnormal shape may be lopsided (asymmetric) or split in two (double). Sometimes you may not find out about this anomaly until you undergo an HSG, since this situation would not be recognized during a routine pelvic exam. But since the majority of women with this disorder have related urinary tract problems, chances are the situation was noted before you decided to conceive.

One of the more common disorders of fusion is the septate uterus. About 3% of women are born with a central ridge (septum) made of tissue that splits the uterus in two. This birth defect increases the risk of miscarriage and premature delivery. Can it easily be corrected? Yes, if miscarriage becomes an issue. Your RE may be able to remove the ridge through hysteroscopy repair microsurgery, which has replaced the traditional abdominal procedure (the Strassman operation). A successful pregnancy may follow if no other factors exist. On one occasion I spoke to a woman with a double uterus undergoing IVF. In her case, embryos were being transferred into each chamber, doubling the odds of success.

In the case of a single ovary and a working uterus, your doctor may prescribe Clomid or Pergonal in order to ensure the monthly production of an egg. Even if your ovaries don't produce eggs at all (Turner's syndrome or ovarian dysgenesis), you still have the option of carrying a nonbiological child through pursuing IVF with donor egg.

45. AUTOIMMUNE DYSFUNCTION Part a) Sperm Antibodies (Immunoglobulins): What can I do to counteract the fact that my body's antibodies are strangling sperm before they can fertilize any ova? It turns out that I am "allergic" to my husband's sperm. I am appalled. I never realized that my body was capable of developing its own form of birth control.

Ever since the AIDS epidemic took hold in the 1980s, it has raised our consciousness about how we rely on our autoimmune systems for good health. Essentially our bodies produce special immune cells (antibodies) to guard against unwanted intruders related to illness. So it is a revelation to discover that sometimes these "guard" cells may become overzealous in their protective urges and work against our best efforts to get pregnant. Certainly I was taken aback to find that all the months I was working with an ovulation kit to maximize the chance of getting pregnant, my body was working at cross purposes by producing antibodies that were choking my husband's sperm.

What causes these amazingly tough proteins to attack sperm? Antibodies' main function is to defend the body against foreign invasion by infection. When sperm are mistaken for foreign invaders, the antibodies take aim and deactivate the intruders. Lurking in the cervical mucus or bloodstream, they may immobilize sperm, prevent them from proceeding into the uterus, or cause them to clump together. Despite evidence that this form of internal self-defense may interfere with conception, the motivation for this mistaken identity remains a mystery.

Sperm antibodies are not just found in the female population. Men produce sperm antibodies as well, especially following vasectomies. Once the ejaculatory duct is blocked, the sperm die off internally and release a protein into the body. This "intruder" triggers a chain reaction that puts antibodies on the defensive.

By now you may be wondering why you ever used birth control, but remember that your body's defenses change over time—even from cycle to cycle. Chances are that you were not producing antibodies during a time in your life when you weren't ready to start a family, so you don't need to harbor any self-recriminations about precautions you took. Women whose partners used condoms may have protected themselves against pelvic inflammatory disease (PID), which is responsible for the prevalence of tubal damage among the infertile population. Using condoms may have suppressed the antibody response as well.

After antibodies have been identified, your RE will determine which of three types you have and how they attack the sperm. Do they grab the head, the tail, or in between? The best scenario seems to be the tail, which rules out antibodies as a factor. Otherwise you will have to consider further measures, such as IUI or IVF in order to bypass the antibodies. If the antibodies are mainly congregating in the mucus, intrauterine insemination may be the simplest solution. Success rate ranges from 20 to 40% per IUI attempt, depending upon the level of antibodies in the genital tract. With IVF, micromanipulation and other modifications in the petri dish may enhance the outcome.

If the antibodies are suspected to be at the root of recurrent pregnancy loss, your RE may prescribe a daily course of prednisone, a steroid, to reduce the levels of antibodies. Or you may want to explore more experimental treatments, such as heparin or baby aspirin therapy. An immunophenotype—a new, expensive (more than $1,000) workup test to measure specific antibodies (killer cells)—can determine whether you are a candidate for immune therapy. In extreme cases, intravenous immunoglobulin (IVIG) may be recommended. Even specialists who are skeptical about this treatment acknowledge that aspirin and heparin could have a tonic effect for patients with high levels of antiphospholipid antibodies (APAs) although for reasons not entirely understood. In my own case the levels of antibodies dwindled after I altered my diet and turned to daily meditation.

See: *Autoimmune dysfunction part b*

Part b) Miscarriages: What treatments exist to help me avoid miscarriage caused by my immune system? There appears to be something amiss with my immune system that triggers it to reject a pregnancy as a foreign body. After two miscarriages I'm nervous about conceiving again. I have heard about a new, experimental treatment that involves blood transfusions, which sounds a little worrisome.

How autoimmune factors may influence the outcome of a pregnancy is a hotly debated topic. Since reproductive immunology is the subspecialty of the moment, the medical community has not yet devised a standard about what levels indicate a problem and how to proceed on the basis of test results. The patient is in a quandary: The very same test results deemed normal by one doctor may cause the next specialist to recommend a course of blood transfusions. Sometimes the art of ART may lead the practitioner to suggest treatments based on observations rather than on clinical evidence.

In an effort to identify causes for what may be going wrong for the 20% of "unexplained" fertility cases, the immune system is the focus of reproductive medical researchers. The dilemma boils down to this: Why do some couples produce high-quality embryos that fail to implant properly in the uterus? A small group of experts believe that perhaps over one third of the unexplained category may find the answer to their implantation failure by looking at autoimmune dysfunction as the reason for failed embryo implantation. Yet even among this small cadre of immunologists there is great divergence on proper treatment of the problem.

As we all know, the central function of our immune system is to protect the body from disease. When bacteria enter your body, the immune system sends out white blood cells to create antibodies that attempt to combat the illness. If such antibodies reject a pregnancy, you may have an autoimmune disorder. Under optimal circumstances, a woman's immune system acknowledges the embryo and creates bodyguards (antileukocyte or blocking antibodies) to keep it safe during the first half of gestation. Without a strong defense line of blockers, the threat of miscarriage becomes greater. According to recent studies, one third of women suffering from multiple miscarriage have tested positive for an autoimmune syndrome.

Any of four autoimmune dysfunctions may be interfering with a full-term pregnancy: (1) antinuclear antibodies (ANAs), (2) antiphospholipid antibodies (APAs), (3) antithyroid antibodies (ATAs), and (4) lupuslike anticoagulant.

ANAs: In this scenario, antibodies attack the basic cell proteins of the fertilized egg, like its DNA. Women who are prone to inflammatory diseases, such as rheumatoid arthritis, are likely to fall into this category. Steroids (prednisone) may be prescribed together with an anticoagulant (heparin) as an antidote.

APAs: Since these antibodies prevent implantation by cutting off the blood supply to the placenta, they are the focus of intensive research. Heparin with baby aspirin and/or blood transfusions may be indicated.

ATAs: Hypothyroidism, caused by antibodies attacking the thyroid gland, may be counteracted by daily medication.

Statistics from Pacific Fertility Medical Centers for ART, one of the leaders in researching this subspecialty, show high levels of APAs in nearly half its patients with chronic PID and two thirds of those with endometriosis. Their team assigns the bulk of the blame on antiphospholipid antibodies, which may be undermining normal placenta development. Good placenta function is dependent upon support from phospholipids, which hold it in place and ensure sufficient blood flow between mother and fetus. The implication, which has stirred much debate, is that a high level of APAs may set off a negative chain reaction that creates blood clots in the placenta, resulting in early pregnancy loss. However, as of this writing, this theory remains controversial and is not widely supported within the field of reproductive medicine.

If your APA blood test reads positive in two consecutive cycles, and no other obvious factors have been identified, you may be concerned that an incipient autoimmune syndrome may put a future pregnancy at risk. Could antiphospholipid antibodies be working as built-in birth control by preventing embryos from ever developing beyond a few days? A small group of experts suspect this to be the case. Miscarriage is technically the failure of a fetus to implant properly. But if the antibodies throw off blood clots within days of conception, implantation failure may be harder to detect.

Could this mean that a late period is actually a lost pregnancy? This has always been a popular suspicion among infertile women. A full screening for eight phospholipids (21 markers) is recommended in this case to determine if APAs may be a factor. The standard antidote is low-dose baby or adult aspirin and heparin, an anticoagulant. Although the aspirin crosses to the baby, there is no evidence in all its years of use that low-dose aspirin contributes to birth defects. This treatment is also indicated for women with lupus erythematosus.

In cases of alloimmunity, where a woman's body is "allergic" to her partner's sperm, an extremely controversial treatment has been introduced in recent years that involves a course of immunization with the white blood cells of her partner (or that of a male donor). In order to build antileukocyte (ALA) levels, this protocol requires treatment every four to six weeks until delivery. By having the man's white blood cells injected into the woman's body, in theory she maintains the level of maternal blocking antibodies required for good embryo implantation.

Another experimental procedure, intravenous immunoglobulin (IVIG) therapy, may be suggested. In this case a transfusion every four to six weeks is recommended to keep up ALA levels and protect the pregnancy throughout the term. Of course, before you make this commitment, you have to address the risks involved in transfusions (adverse reactions, bacteria, etc.) to both mother and baby.

46. BACTERIA: How do I find out if my problem is a vaginal bacterial infection? I have heard that it is possible to become temporarily infertile as the result of a mild vaginal bacterial infection, which is cured very simply with antibiotics.

The jury is still out on whether bacteria caused by vaginitis play a major role in the drama of infertility.

Certainly, if the vaginal climate is not receptive to sperm, how can you expect to conceive? It's also clear that the discharge associated with infection may stop sperm in its tracks too early along the reproductive route. What's really frightening is the epidemic of chlamydia, now the leading cause of PID. Only 30% of the infected population has been diagnosed and treated, while the majority of carriers manifest no symptoms until the damage has been done to their reproductive abilities. Also threatening to fertility are mycoplasma and some types of anaerobic bacteria, which may lurk in the reproductive passages.

How do you get infected? Possibilities abound. The obvious way is through unprotected sexual contact, and that is why condoms are the preferred mode of birth control these days. Early designs of the IUD also invited bacteria into the reproductive tract. A revolutionary theory postulates that bacteria may even be transmitted during childbirth from the mother.

If you suspect that you have a silent infection, your RE will take a Pap smear to culture you for moniliasis (yeast) and trichomoniasis, a sexually transmitted disease. Perhaps 15% of sexually active men are believed to be carrying the trichomonas bug unbeknownst to them. For women, the obvious signal of a problem is a change in the color or quantity of vaginal discharge. A strong oral antibiotic may be indicated to cure this situation. More common are yeast infections, which may be caused by something as innocent as wearing panty hose; synthetic fibers may raise the temperature in the crotch and encourage bacteria to grow. Treatment may include a regimen of suppositories, antibiotics, and a diet rich in yogurt.

Currently, the main suspect in the field of fertility is mycoplasma, hostile microorganisms in the genital tract that may attack sperm and negatively impact on motility. An aggressive course of tetracycline may clear up this condition. On the downside, antibiotics may trigger a yeast infection. In order to protect against this, your doctor may recommend suppositories.

See: PID

47. CERVICAL MUCUS DYSFUNCTION: Part a) Is there anything I can do to change the consistency of my cervical mucus? During my workup it was diagnosed as being too "thin." This is the first time in my life that being described as thin has bothered me.

Ideally, for you to get pregnant your cervical mucus must provide a welcome environment for healthy, active sperm as they enter the reproductive system. Mucus is generated by glands in the cervical canal, which connects the uterus to the outer cervical opening. At the time of ovulation, "friendly" mucus will appear transparent and stretchy to the touch. You may experience it as a clear vaginal discharge. It should be free of bacteria or antibodies and abundant enough to propel the sperm along its way to the egg. After ovulation its consistency thickens as the transport function shuts down.

Cervical mucus serves a dual purpose: In addition to propelling the sperm toward the fallopian tubes, it prepares the sperm to fertilize an egg by encouraging the release of enzymes (capacitation). To keep momentum, it must be free of antibodies and other hostile invaders. When the mucus fails on either count, a fertility problem arises. And this situation is not uncommon: For an estimated one in 15 patients the diagnosis is cervical mucus insufficiency.

What causes a lack of mucus? Possible reasons include infection, antibodies, and hormonal or other chemical imbalances caused by exposure to medications such as DES. Strangely, clomiphene citrate (the fertility pill) may diminish the production of cervical mucus if taken several cycles in a row and must be discontinued in such cases. In most patients levels will return to normal within one cycle.

See: Chlamydia, DES, cough syrup

Part b) Cervical Infections/Mycoplasma: If I've had cervicitis in the past, could it have caused permanent damage? I have read that there is an organism that exists in either the cervix or semen that may act as a built-in form of birth control. How do I find out if this is my problem?

In trying to explain why so many couples suffer from "unexplained" infertility, experts are examining the reproductive tract for booby traps. Since the cervix is positioned at the entry of the reproductive tract, it is especially susceptible to attack by bacteria or sexually transmitted diseases. Almost any activity may irritate cervical tissue: the effort of childbirth, hormone medications (including birth control pills), even sexual intercourse. Sometimes a chronic inflammation, cervicitis, may be so mild as to be unnoticeable. The tip-off may be symptoms like backache, spotting, and urinary problems. Once you begin to notice excess vaginal discharge, you know there's trouble.

With pelvic inflammatory disease (PID) on the rise, the most likely causes of cervicitis include sexually transmitted diseases and certain bacteria. If gonorrhea is ruled out, mycoplasma may be the next suspect. A hostile microorganism, mycoplasma has been known to ambush sperm in the cervical mucus and counteract embryo implantation. Since it may do damage insidiously and silently, you may not have a clue that you have an infection until you have trouble conceiving. In fact, you and your partner may be passing the infection back and forth.

When infection erodes the cervical tissue, complications like ulcers or polyps may arise. Erosion may be corrected with an application of silver nitrate or by electrocautery, depending on the extent of damage. In the case of polyps—small protrusions—the RE may be able to remove them during an office visit. Advanced cases will require dilation and curettage (D&C). To rule out cancer, the doctor may take a biopsy in addition to a Pap smear. How can you get a diagnosis? Both you and your partner need to get a bacterial culture analysis. After a course of antibiotics you will be analyzed again to be sure that indeed you have conquered this infection.

See: Bacteria, chlamydia

48. DIETHYLSTILBESTROL (DES): *How can I, a DES daughter, find out more about my prospects for childbearing? I recently found out that my mother took DES when she was carrying me and that this drug could have negative repercussions on my fertility. My uterus was unable to hold an IUD, and now I am worried that I won't be able to carry a baby to term. . . . My mother-in-law took DES when she was pregnant with my husband. Will his sperm be affected?*

Unfortunately, the legacy for DES daughters born between 1943 and the late 1950s is often a permanently altered cervix and possibly a uterus that may be resistant to estrogen. Because of exposure to an artificial substance in the placenta at some point when they were in the womb, these women may not be able to carry a pregnancy. Additional estrogen will not act as a cure.

Most gynecologists are familiar with the range of DES reproductive disorders, beginning with cervical abnormalities. Where DES affected the structure of the cervix, one early symptom may be abnormal mucus production that diminishes sperm motility. Secondly, an HSG may reveal a T-shaped uterus with an abnormally small cavity, another hallmark symptom. If you are unable to sustain an IUD because you have an odd-shaped uterus, you may have been exposed to DES. An unreceptive endometrial lining may offer another clue. Even when DES daughters ovulate regularly and exhibit good estrogen production, their endometria are unable to support an embryo, and they experience miscarriage. Development of the fallopian tubes usually remains unaffected, although sometimes their length exceeds the norm.

Although repair surgery doesn't apply to this diagnosis since the drug exposure damaged the intrinsic nature of the tissue, ART offers other options. Treatment for DES women falls under the category of cervical factor. Generally, intrauterine insemination (IUI) is indicated in order to bypass the hostile mucus. Since the uterus may be small or T-shaped, the concern after conception is to take precautions against an incompetent cervix. Taking a stitch in the cervix (cerclage) after the first trimester can hold the pregnancy in place. Ironically, the very drug that was designed to prevent miscarriage in the mother has vastly increased just that possibility for the daughter.

For men, DES exposure is manifested through reduced sperm counts. Nearly one third of DES sons have exhibited syndromes of the urogenital tract, ranging from benign epididymal cysts to infertility. Varicoceles, the varicose veins that interfere with sperm production, are another common symptom of DES exposure. Again, the new ICSI (single sperm injection) procedure that is part of most IVF programs may become the standard solution to problems of low sperm count.

49. DIET: Can my fertile days be impaired or enhanced by what I eat or drink?

You are what you eat, as the old saying goes. In this case, consider yourself in training not unlike an athlete. For optimal fertility you might want to modify your diet and eliminate potentially harmful elements. Whatever you do, this is not the time to go on a full-fledged diet; weight loss may interfere with the delicate flow of hormone production so crucial to success. Even as little as five pounds one way or the other may create a problem.

The rule of thumb with diet is to be good to yourself yet to exercise common sense. Avoid alcohol and other recreational substances while you're trying to conceive. Also off limits are meats and poultry that may carry additional estrogen, which may alter your levels. Try to incorporate more soy foods into your meals. If you can handle the implications, treat yourself as if you were pregnant and take this opportunity to improve your diet even to the extent of taking prenatal vitamins.

Quite possibly the nature of your uterine lining may be affected by your intake. The one universally recognized culprit is caffeine; too much coffee is considered a precursor of miscarriage. Basically no more than 300 mg per day (about three cups of non-Starbucks coffee or four cans of soda) are recommended. If you can make the switch to Japanese green tea, some doctors advise it.

What about smoking? Current studies show conflicting results. The Center for Reproductive Research and Testing in Rockville, Maryland, cites negative impact on the uterine linings in women who smoke more than

16 cigarettes a day. The University of Toronto observes that smoking delays implantation. Yet other studies have not found any connection between smoking and infertility.

50. ENDOMETRIOSIS: Should I anticipate any trouble conceiving as a result of my medical history of endometriosis? At age 30 I was diagnosed with endometriosis after experiencing painful periods. I had surgery to correct this problem. Now, three years later, I am getting married. . . . ADENOMYOSIS: After experiencing severe cramps with my period, I was diagnosed with adenomyosis. I understand that this means that endometrial tissue is growing into the uterine wall. I want to have it corrected, but will this reduce my chances of getting pregnant? I am 39.

Endometriosis, formerly known as the "career woman's disease," affects an estimated 10% of American women between the ages of 15 and 49. Ongoing menstruation without a sustained pregnancy may contribute to the prevalence of this condition, which is characterized by painful periods, irregular bleeding, and infertility. Some women, who may have no physical symptoms at all, learn of this diagnosis when they have difficulty conceiving. Other women previously diagnosed may have no trouble at all conceiving. The ability to conceive may depend on how advanced the case is.

Basically, this condition is caused by endometrial cells growing outside their proper place in the uterus. These cells may develop into adhesions that attach to other parts of the reproductive organs (ovaries, bladder, intestine, or abdominal wall). Depending on size, growths are described as implants (small patches), nodules, or endometriomas ("chocolate" cysts). Cysts range in size from a pea to a grapefruit. In advanced cases of endometriosis, adhesions may crisscross the pelvis and bind the uterus, fallopian tubes, and ovaries to one another.

The doctor will score the case on a range of one to 15, indicating a diagnosis of mild to severe. The disorder may begin in one of two ways. Either some backwash of menstrual blood releases endometrial cells into the pelvis, or the immune system isn't reacting to clear these unwanted cells from implanting in the wrong place. If the endometrial tissue embeds into the uterine wall, the diagnosis changes to *adenomyosis*. Symptoms are related to the uterus, which becomes enlarged, tender, and slightly inflamed.

Can giving birth when you're under 30 help you avoid this syndrome? If there is no history of this disease in your family, a sustained pregnancy might reduce the occurrence. However, since the disease is genetic, if your mother or sisters have been diagnosed, odds are greater that you will follow suit even if you have a baby.

How can you find out if you have endometriosis? Once a cyst bursts or leaks blood, the sudden pain will alert you to the problem. Another common symptom is discomfort during intercourse: Pressure on a nodule or scar tissue can cause discomfort, which will tip you off. Sometimes your gynecologist will notice nodules or an enlarged ovary during a routine physical exam. A laparoscopy may follow so that the doctor can see the extent of the adhesions. During this procedure the doctor may remove some of the tissue to alleviate blockage. Follow-up treatment includes oral contraceptives, danazol, gonadotropin-releasing hormone (GnRH) analogs, and progestins.

51. ENVIRONMENT: Could either pollution or pesticides be a factor in preventing me from getting pregnant? Sometimes I feel that the air I breathe is polluted and poisonous. I worry about pesticides in my food and have read articles that confirm my fears.

Most infertility is diagnosed as a result of other factors, but our environment and the food we eat must be taken into consideration when approaching any health issue. Preliminary research supports the popular notion that pollutants do play a role in our reproductive health as well as in our general well-being. In 1996 Resolve, the national fertility network, participated in a conference that explored the effects of estrogen mimics (dioxins and DDT) commonly found in the world around us. Evidence seems to be building that exposure to these substances does have a negative impact on fertility for all living creatures. If the connection between chemicals and cancer has been made, we can expect that other disorders will follow.

Easily identifiable toxins have come under suspicion regarding infertility in recent times. Why is endometriosis so widespread in the United States? While there is no definitive answer, one 1993 study points to dioxin exposure as a factor. By suppressing the immune system, dioxins (including PCB compounds and X rays) may suppress normal hormonal production. Miscarriage is also more likely due to dioxin overexposure, according to this study. Although this opinion is not universally held, experts do agree that a compromised immune system is at the crux of endometriosis.

Other prime suspects in the realm of irregular menstruation are common chemical compounds associated with modern life, such as dry-cleaning fluids and paint thinners. Benzene exposure may wreak havoc on ovulation as well. And brace yourself for this popular suspect on the short list: nail polish. Could the proliferation of nail salons in the 1990s actually be keeping women infertile? It might be worth going manicureless for a few cycles to find out.

See: Endometriosis

52. FALLOPIAN TUBES (DISORDERS) Part a) Hydrosalpinx: Is it possible to contract a tubal infection without symptoms? In a recent HSG blockage was identified. My doctor found an abnormal distension of my tubes because of inflammation (hydrosalpinx). He explained that an infection may have compromised the interior of my tube (endothelial lining). I have been married for eight years and using a diaphragm. I never felt any discomfort, and nothing showed up on my Pap smears. Could my diaphragm be the culprit?

For one in three women facing infertility, tubal disease will be her diagnosis. What is the reason for this widespread female health crisis? Heading the list is pelvic inflammatory disease (PID), a general term for sexually transmitted infections of the reproductive tract that flare up into inflammations and leave behind scar tissue. With multiple sexual partners the norm today, an upsurge in venereal diseases has become a public health issue.

Some of the bacteria responsible for tubal disease may enter the body silently, coming to light only when you don't get pregnant after a year of trying. And, yes, bacteria may have entered your body through diaphragm use. Perhaps you left it in place too long, or it wasn't perfectly antiseptic. Any action that alters the environment of your uterus, including douching, may invite a serious infection without manifesting any outward signs.

Past abdominal surgery for appendicitis or peritonitis may create tubal distortion. Once the tube's shape is constricted, egg and sperm may not be able to rendezvous successfully, and a fertility problem ensues. *Hydrosalpinges* are distortions of the fimbria, the fringed part of the tube that connects to the ovary. Once an infection causes these fringes to become glued together, they may form a sac. The natural fluids within the tube then become trapped and create a water balloon–like sac. Eventually, the pressure of the balloon erodes the quality of the tubal lining and compromises its structure. Depending on how the hydrosalpinx is graded, it may be curable with surgery. When the patient is under 35, the RE will be more apt to recommend a repair procedure.

While Pap smears may catch advanced cases of PID, others go unnoticed for years. Not everyone who has been treated for a venereal disease develops blockage, but some women who were not aware of infections will discover blockage during workups. Now you may be struggling with the notion that your birth control may have left you with a fertility problem. But even if it did, the reason doesn't matter anymore. What matters is the plan of action you as a couple need to develop with your doctor at this time in order to realize your goal.

Getting a diagnosis is your license to look into the future instead of dwelling on the past and what you might have done differently. Take advantage of the technology women of the twenty-first century are fortunate enough to have. In order to build our families, we may have to let go of the simple notions that led us to this point in our adult lives and turn to medical science. If you find it difficult to let go of guilt feelings or self-recriminations, ask your reproductive endocrinologist for a referral to a psychologist with a specialty in this area. Short-term counseling may help you put these thoughts to rest so that you can focus your energies on moving ahead.

See: Chlamydia, HSG

Part b) Opening Surgically: Can appendicitis create infertility—or harm my fallopian tubes? After a case of appendicitis (or peritonitis) several years ago, my doctor told me that there was some scarring of my tubes as a result. I've heard that laser surgery is quite simple in this case.

Tubal factor accounts for the diagnosis in more than one of three female infertility patients. Scarred or damaged tubes may result either from a chronic condition like endometriosis or from an acute infection caused by a sexually transmitted disease (STD). With the "silent" STD chlamydia now the number one infectious disease, according to 1995 figures from the Centers for Disease Control and Prevention, the issue of "safe" sex takes on new implications. Since chlamydia has never before been tracked, its ranking ahead of gonorrhea and AIDS has serious repercussions in the reproductive arena especially because it is considered a primary cause of infertility and complications during pregnancy.

The fallopian tubes, the hollow, curved vessels that connect the ovary to the uterus, act as the meeting place along the sperm's route to find the egg. As the egg leaves the ovary, the delicate "fingers" of the fallopian tube (fimbriae) guide it through to the uterus. For up to five days the egg wends its way down into the uterus, where it implants on the wall. Fertilization typically occurs in the distal part of the tube, farthest from the uterus. Problems arise from damaged fimbriae or from scar tissue anywhere along the tubal path.

Blockage may occur at either end of the tube: close to the uterus (proximal) or close to the ovary (distal).

The better prognosis will be related to a proximal blockage. Either situation may be the result of a local inflammation (i.e., pelvic inflammatory disease, appendicitis, bowel ailment) or of scar tissue caused by endometriosis. Since these conditions may occur painlessly, the first clue you may have of a problem is the inability to conceive. A tubal (ectopic) pregnancy is another clue that scar tissue has developed around the tubes and trapped an embryo. The part of the workup that explores tubal function—hysterosalpingogram or laparoscopy—determines where blockage exists and whether both tubes are affected.

Depending upon your age and the extent and location of tubal damage, your reproductive endocrinologist may recommend in vitro over repair surgery for best results. Data collected by the American Medical Association support the conclusion that IVF is more effective than repair surgery. If the situation requires removing scar tissue from around the tubes, the natural pregnancy rate may approach 50% under the best of circumstances. Correcting distal blockage (hydrosalpinx) has a success rate between 15 and 30% depending upon the degree of damage versus an 18 to 20% IVF success.

For women under 35, doctors will be more likely to evaluate whether the damage is correctable through microsurgery. After all, the younger the patient, the higher the risk of multiple pregnancy through IVF. These ambulatory procedures are generally performed laparoscopically, through the belly button, leaving no external scar. What is so difficult about reopening the tubes? Especially in these days of zapping obstructions with laser beams? The problem is that scar tissue often grows back almost immediately, perhaps before your next cycle, taking you right back to square one with blocked tubes. Secondly, damaged tubes enhance the risk of an ectopic (tubal) pregnancy. An embryo lodged in the fallopian tube may lead to a rupture, internal bleeding, and a life-threatening situation for you.

See: *Hysterosalpingogram, Laparoscopy*

53. FIBROID TUMORS: How can I find out if my fibroids are preventing me from conceiving? Since the age of 18 I have known of small fibroids on my uterus. When they were first identified, my gynecologist assured me that they should not interfere with a full-term pregnancy. Now, 15 years later, one of my friends is having a myomectomy to remove her fibroids at her doctor's suggestion so that she can try to get pregnant.

If you have been told that you have fibroid tumors, you are not alone. Nearly one quarter of the American female population of childbearing years develops these benign growths, according to the latest statistics from the AMA. For black women the incidence of fibroids is three times higher than among white women. Chances are if your mother or sister has fibroids and you are over 30, then you are next. Yet despite its widespread reach, fibroids are responsible for infertility in fewer than 4% of cases.

Thankfully, two out of three cases are completely asymptomatic. In other words, you may live your entire life without even recognizing that you have fibroids. The hallmark symptom is excessive menstrual bleeding, followed by acute pelvic pain or pressure. Prolonged bleeding may be due to a change in the size of the fibroid or to the pressure that the mass is exerting on the uterine lining (endometrium). An increase in estrogen levels, caused by birth control pills, hormone therapy, or pregnancy, may result in a sudden enlargement.

What are fibroids? They are muscle tissue gone haywire. They range in size from the extremes of a pea (2 cm) to a grapefruit (20 cm) and tend to develop in clusters. For some undetermined reason they spin off from the wall of the uterus (myometrium) to create lumps or masses. They thrive on estrogen and so they may grow during pregnancy, when estrogen levels are high, and shrink after menopause, as hormone levels fall. Certainly the presence of an "abnormal" growth on your reproductive organs that is sometimes referred to as a "tumor" is unsettling. But rest assured that it is not cancer; a mere one in every 10,000 women with fibroids is diagnosed with uterine cancer, and most often these patients are past childbearing years.

Depending on where they appear, fibroids fall into three subgroups. Most often they appear on the outside covering of the uterus (subserous), which is the most benign location. The second most common place they occur is in the uterine wall (intramural). A small number of fibroids also develop under the uterine lining itself (submucosal). Because of their location, this last category is most likely to trigger a fertility problem.

Complications become more likely if the fibroid grows in the interior of the uterus. The submucosal fibroid may prevent fertilization either by blocking the tubes or by altering the quality of the uterine wall so that the fertilized egg cannot implant. Even if implantation is successful, a badly placed fibroid may cause miscarriage as it increases in size as the result of the increase in female hormone levels. Or it may compete with the embryo for space in the uterus. Removal is usually the recommended treatment via hysteroscopic microsurgery, when possible. For deeper-seated fibroids, a laparotomy (abdominal surgery) may be indicated. When performed by an experienced RE, this repair should not compromise uterine function.

See: *Estrogen, HSG, Miscarriage, Painful periods*

54. HORMONAL IMBALANCES Part a) Prolactin (Galactorrhea): How can I regulate my lactation hormones? It appears that an imbalance in the production of prolactin, a mammary gland hormone, is creating an ovulation problem for me. I am in my late thirties.

Ironically, the pituitary may throw off the regular course of ovulation by secreting excess prolactin, the hormone that stimulates milk production after childbirth. A blood test can determine whether the levels are too high, or you may even notice your nipples leaking a milky substance. This imbalance is often associated with polycystic ovarian syndrome (PCOS).

How can your body play such a cruel trick? Faulty pituitary function is the culprit. Sometimes a small, benign tumor (adenoma) forms on the pituitary and interferes with proper prolactin production. Generally, such a tumor responds well to drug therapy so that surgery is indicated only if the adenoma is large (over 10 mm). Or prolactin-producing cells may become hyperactive because of developments in the thyroid, kidney, or adrenal gland. Prescription drugs (tranquilizers, painkillers, contraceptives) have also been found to affect levels adversely. Alcohol and recreational drugs may also stimulate prolactin levels.

The antidote to this condition, bromocriptine (Parlodel), suppresses this runaway function by working to shrink the adenoma and control levels. Better than 85% of patients with this diagnosis respond well to treatment with Parlodel, which comes in both tablet and capsule forms. If no other mitigating factors complicate the situation, such women may go on to conceive naturally.

Parlodel does have some serious side effects, ranging from headaches, stuffy nose, and vomiting to possible high blood pressure, dizziness, or even fainting. If you have a severe reaction, your doctor will lower the dosage. In any case, you should refrain from driving or operating machinery until you have a handle on how you feel.

Part b) Luteal Phase Defect: Is there anything that can be done to compensate for the LH factor in my case?

If the end of your cycle falls under 12 days and blood tests confirm low levels of progesterone, you may have a luteal phase defect. In other words, your endometrial lining is not being primed to receive the fertilized egg for gestation.

The second half of your menstrual cycle (the luteal phase) begins when your pituitary releases luteinizing hormone (LH) in order to trigger ovulation. Once the follicle releases an egg, the empty shell (corpus luteum) turns yellow. In this form, it pumps female hormones (estrogen and progesterone) into the bloodstream in anticipation of a pregnancy. If an embryo implants, the corpus luteum remains in place during the first trimester and keeps estrogen and progesterone levels up to support the growing fetus.

A luteal phase defect (LPD) reveals itself in the way the endometrial lining responds to ovulation. While the follicle develops in the ovary, the lining should be growing thicker in anticipation of its nurturing role to come. After ovulation, the corpus luteum takes over in preparing the lining. Low levels of progesterone and other key nutrients would indicate that something is amiss in this delicate operation. Occasionally fertility drug treatment may artificially create an LPD factor, which can be adjusted chemically. More often signals are getting crossed at ovulation time.

If your RE suspects an LPD factor to be your diagnosis, your blood levels will need to be closely monitored. A reading under 10 nanograms per milliliter of progesterone confirms a problem. Next, an endometrial biopsy will be scheduled following ovulation (provided no pregnancy is detected). Depending upon your age, fertility drug therapy beginning with Clomid may be indicated to adjust levels and compensate for the deficit. Supplemental progesterone may be added to the protocol, along with estrogen.

For women over 35 an LH factor may be an early symptom of ovarian shutdown. As you approach menopause, the latter part of your cycle shortens. A thorough workup will determine if this is happening to your body. In this case, use of donor eggs may be a more hopeful route.

55. INTRAUTERINE DEVICE (IUD): *How can I find out if my IUD may have caused some permanent damage? For many years I used an IUD to prevent an unwanted pregnancy. Now I am ready to start a family.*

Theoretically the IUD seemed to offer a safe birth control option without the use of drugs. The concept has been around for centuries: Insert a foreign object (in this case a piece of plastic or metal) in the uterus to prevent pregnancy until you are ready to start a family. The foreign body then triggers the appearance of cells (macrophages), which consume the fertilized egg prior to implantation—a sound theory.

But for some women—especially for those who were using the Dalkon Shield—the IUD legacy may have worked too well at keeping pregnancy at bay. This particular model is characterized by a string that threads from the uterus through the cervix and into the vaginal canal. Unfortunately, the string may have acted as a conduit for bacteria to enter the reproductive system and set the stage for pelvic inflammatory disease (PID) and widespread adhesions throughout the area. Since users didn't expect to get pregnant while the IUD was in place, finding out that its repercussions might be long term was a rude awakening.

Is potential damage limited to the Dalkon Shield? No, sad to say. Bacteria may have entered the pelvis during the insertion of any brand of IUD. Even during IUD removal the uterus or cervix may undergo irreversible trauma or scarring that may persistently interfere with embryo implantation. Typically PID in IUD users affects just one fallopian tube; that may mean that natural conception is still possible. Of course the IUD did not compromise every user's fertility. I have personal knowledge of one woman who actually managed to get pregnant while her IUD was in place and another who conceived two children naturally after removal of the Dalkon Shield.

56. MALE FACTOR—UNDERWEAR: *Is it true that tight Jockey shorts can act as a form of birth control by inhibiting sperm production?*

Although there is no conclusive evidence on this subject, studies have been conducted to measure whether underwear styles have any effect on sperm. Since it is a fact that the scrotum should be cooler than the rest of the body for optimal production, it would seem to follow that constricting underwear could interfere with effective production. At the 1996 ASRM convention, one study reported no difference in scrotal temperature or semen quality between a group of men wearing Jockey shorts and another in boxers. Since men with enlarged varicoceles may have higher scrotal temperatures, boxer shorts may cool the area. But if a structural problem or bacterial infection is impeding sperm production, a change in underwear style won't help.

57. MISCARRIAGE: Is there anything I can do to help ensure that I can carry my next pregnancy to term and not miscarry again? I had a miscarriage last year and haven't conceived again during the past 10 months. I am worried about losing another pregnancy. . . . MATERNAL MISCARRIAGE: My mother lost a couple of pregnancies between me and my sister. Are there hereditary implications?

The emotional toll of losing a pregnancy can create repercussions as you try to conceive again. Sadly, it's a commonplace event. Of course you question any actions that may be at the root of the miscarriage. Where did I go wrong? Did I use too much hair spray? Physically, did I overdo it somehow? The answer to all the above is no, it's not your fault. Not even infections have been linked to recurrent miscarriage. The only known factors that may cause pregnancy loss are smoking and drinking, and since we all have met women who smoked and drank during pregnancy yet still produced healthy babies, even that one drink or cigarette you had before you realized you were pregnant would not have made the difference.

Experts estimate that miscarriage affects about one in five clinically detectable pregnancies within the first 20 weeks of gestation. Typically a miscarriage occurs around Week 8 with the subsequent bleeding around Week 12. More than half these first trimester losses are due to chromosomal abnormalities (aneuploidies), which also means increased risk for the woman over

40. The balance of losses results from a problem with carrying the pregnancy that could be related to structural, hormonal, or immunological issues. Although they may be able to conceive on their own, the couple who experience multiple miscarriages are considered to have an infertility problem.

Chances of miscarriage are 33% if you're over 40, 18% if you're between 35 and 39, 12% for early thirties, and 10% for late twenties. If you've lost one pregnancy, your risk may increase slightly with your second pregnancy. Once you've lost two pregnancies, the risk more than doubles with your third. For example, if you are 31, your initial odds were 12%, then 16% the second time, and up to 38% on round three if you lost both pregnancies. Because of this escalation of the odds, the American College of Obstetrics and Gynecologists now suggests testing following two losses in order to protect the third pregnancy.

To determine if your diagnosis is related to a chromosomal issue, the doctor will need to analyze blood from you and your partner and, if possible, from the fetal tissue. As a rule, your doctor will recommend this course if you've had more than two early miscarriages. If results show that either or both of you have an abnormal karyotype (chromosomal profile), you may want to consider donor gametes (eggs/sperm).

The second leading reason for miscarriage is a hormonal deficit, most often a lack of progesterone in the second half of the cycle (luteal phase defect). During the luteal phase, the uterus prepares to accept embryo implantation by building up the endometrium. An endometrial biopsy taken at the end of a cycle can determine if LPD is the correct diagnosis. When progesterone or estradiol (estrogen) production is low, the problem may lie in a follicular phase deficiency. Possibly, the corpus luteum (empty follicle) is not priming the endometrium sufficiently. Female hormonal imbalances can be diagnosed by blood tests and corrected through medication.

In 15% of miscarriages, doctors will uncover anatomical reasons, such as fibroids, incompetent cervixes, and uterine abnormalities. Most of these abnormalities can be corrected and followed by uneventful, healthy pregnancies. For the remaining four out of 10 cases, immunology may lead to a diagnosis. Blood tests may determine that the woman has developed either an autoimmune syndrome that causes her body to reject the embryo as a foreign body or an alloimmune syndrome that reacts hostilely to the sperm. With proper care there is every good hope of conceiving again and giving birth to a full-term baby.

Depending upon who you are, how long you were trying to conceive and how far along you were may also contribute to how you react to miscarriage. Some women simply shrug it off and determine to try again immediately. Others feel the need to grieve and acknowledge the loss. But taking time out of treatment for any reason may be a luxury if you are over 35 and determined to carry to term. And even a history of miscarriage doesn't rule out a future baby. I have met mothers who have had as many as six previous miscarriages.

See: *Endometrial biopsy, Fibroids*

58. OVULATION DISORDER: *Anovulation (No Ovulation): Can I be treated for the failure of my ovaries to produce an egg in each cycle?*

The key to treatment is to find out why your ovaries aren't functioning properly. Do you have a history of irregular periods? Is your cycle unusually short (under

21 days) or superlong (over 35 days)? Have you gone more than three months without a period (oligomenorrhea)? Or have you stopped menstruating for longer than three months without a pregnancy (amenorrhea)? Sometimes a follicle appears on the ultrasound screen but the egg is not released; this leads to a diagnosis of luteinized unruptured follicle (LUF) syndrome. When LUF is suspected, a follow-up ultrasound after a few days can establish whether the egg was released or not.

Most commonly, ovulation issues are related to disorders of the hypothalamus—the part of the brain that coordinates the release of female hormones into the bloodstream—or of the thyroid gland. Your doctor needs to analyze your hormonal profile through a series of blood tests in order to pinpoint where the disorder lies.

For women over 35, age may be a factor. After that landmark birthday ovulation may become less predictable. Another factor is weight: A sudden loss or gain can interfere with ovarian function. Overweight women may have developed polycystic ovarian syndrome. Symptoms may include hirsutism, the growth of hair on the face or unexpected parts of the body (chest, back, or abdomen). A third possibility is prolactinemia, an elevated level of a protein hormone responsible for producing milk in the mammary glands. White secretion leaking from your nipples may substantiate this diagnosis.

Treatment to stimulate ovulation usually begins with a clomiphene citrate (Clomid) prescription and graduates to human menopausal gonadotropins (Pergonal) where indicated.

59. PERIODS—IRREGULAR OR PAINFUL: *Do severe menstrual cramps indicate a fertility problem? Every 28 days I experience terrible cramps with my period. I have always looked forward to pregnancy as a vacation from this monthly agony. I will be 30 soon and always planned to start my family at that time. What is my prognosis?*

Severe cramps just prior to your period may be a symptom of abnormal activity in the endometrium, caused by either adenomyosis or endometriosis. The former condition is characterized by an enlarged uterus and most often appears in women over 40. Endometriosis occurs when the lining of the uterus (the endometrium) retracts into the reproductive system rather than leaving the body with the usual menstrual flow. Misplaced endometrial tissue may cause scarring and permanent damage to the fallopian tubes.

One effective cure for endometriosis is pregnancy since it suspends hormonal activity for 40 weeks. But the catch-22 is that in advanced cases, you can't conceive because of the tubal blockage caused by endometriosis. Consult your specialist about whether IVF is appropriate in your case. Another exciting breakthrough treatment is the introduction of danazol, a form of testosterone, which has been shown to reverse the damage of endometriosis and allow for natural conception.

Another possible reason for severe cramping is the presence of large fibroids. These growths in the uterine wall can play havoc with your cycle, manifesting as pain in the abdomen and lower back, pressing on the bowels or kidneys, and interfering with these functions. Depending on their location, fibroids may compromise your fertility and need to be removed surgically. If this is your diagnosis and there are no other mitigating factors, you may be able to conceive naturally once they are excised.

See: Endometriosis, Fibroids, IVF

60. PELVIC INFLAMMATORY DISEASE (PID): Is it possible to have a severe PID infection without symptoms? I have a history of yeast infections, which apparently may have been the cause of PID. Now I've learned that my tubes may not be functioning properly as a result of scar tissue. Can the tissue be removed?

Finding out that you have had a serious internal infection without any symptoms is a rude awakening. You may feel that you're being punished for past events that you thought were long buried. I know the feeling; I had them too. Where did things go wrong? At any number of junctures bacteria were introduced into the pelvic area. Countless scenarios offer you the opportunity to worry and flagellate yourself about the past.

Infections may attack any of the reproductive organs: the ovary, the tubes, the endometrium, or the cervix. Possibly complications set in following a miscarriage that you didn't even know about. Sometimes after an abortion or childbirth, nonvenereal bacteria may enter the uterus and spread into the fallopian tubes without any symptoms. Even the IUD is suspect; in its early configuration it acted as a magnet to bacteria creating an inflammation of the fallopian tube (salpingitis).

Could it have been a case of gonorrhea or chlamydia, now the number one public enemy of fertility? Since these conditions are often mistaken for vaginitis, they may wreak havoc inside before being properly diagnosed. Or could it be the result of something as seemingly harmless as douching, which may have compromised the natural defense system? Or did scar tissue form in the pelvis following an appendicitis attack? And on and on.

Regardless of how you ended up with this diagnosis, you must now deal with its impact. You can't undo the damage, but you can take appropriate medical action to get pregnant. Depending on how extensive the damage is, tubal repair is certainly one avenue that needs to be explored. But for the majority of PID cases, the most effective course of action will be IVF.

61. POLYCYSTIC OVARIAN SYNDROME: *I have ovarian cysts that are benign, but how will surgery impact my future chances of having a family? During a routine examination my doctor found that I have ovarian cysts caused by polycystic ovarian syndrome (PCOS) aka Stein-Leventhal syndrome. I am in my early thirties.*

Your ovaries rely on the release of at least one follicle every four to five weeks. When ovulation does not occur on this schedule, a chain of events may develop that could lead to PCOS. If your mother ever developed ovarian cysts, you may have inherited this predisposition. A history of irregular periods or cosmetic concerns like facial hair or chronic acne may be your first clue to this condition. Other common symptoms include diabetes, overactive glands (adrenal, thyroid, or pituitary) or, most often, a weight problem. While obesity is typically associated with this diagnosis approximately half the PCOS population is considerably underweight. Extremes in the levels of fat tissue, insulin, or androgen production can easily topple the proper flow of female hormones necessary to create a viable follicle.

At the root of this problem is abnormal pituitary function that is preventing complete growth of the follicle. When the pituitary doesn't release the proper amounts of female hormones required to make mature follicles (specifically, luteinizing hormone [LH] and follicle-stimulating hormone [FSH]), the immature ones begin to collect in the ovaries. These clusters may develop into small, benign cysts, which do not compromise fertility or require surgical removal. Since the hormone cycle is stuck at the preovulation stage, it may create chronic elevated levels of estrogen and androgen. Over time you will begin to notice symptoms. For example, you may experience irregular bleeding caused by constant estrogen production or facial hair growth resulting from the excess androgen hormone in the bloodstream. In prolonged cases, elevated estrogen levels may possibly cause cancer to develop in the endometrial lining.

How to find out if you have PCOS? A history of irregular periods usually leads to this diagnosis. Upon examination this suspicion will be confirmed if your doctor notices a slight enlargement of the ovaries. Routine blood tests measure all key hormone levels—namely, androgen, LH, FSH, thyroid, and adrenal. Your doctor may also check prolactin levels to complete your hormone profile. Once the diagnosis shows that cysts are present, your doctor will view them via ultrasound. As many as 10 small cysts may appear on each ovary. An endometrial biopsy may be indicated as well to check for cancer in the uterine lining.

Can you combat this condition yourself? If overweight is the issue, you can start there. As long as you create a weight-loss program that includes a simple aerobic activity (walking will do) three times a week, you may be able to gain some control. Select a program that is realistic, and make it part of your regular routine. Getting in shape prior to getting pregnant is a good idea even if you require medical intervention.

To ensure ovulation, your doctor will prescribe fertility drugs. For those patients who do not respond to drug therapy, the doctor may suggest a surgical procedure known as ovarian capsule puncture. Using a laparoscope, the surgeon will use either needle penetration or cautery on several parts of the ovary to regulate ovarian function. In some cases surgical intervention restores monthly ovulation for several cycles.

If none of the above treatments shows results, you may wish to explore in vitro fertilization with your doctor. A new technique is being explored, using immature eggs, that shows promise for women with PCOS. Rather than women using fertility drugs, the small eggs are retrieved vaginally and fertilized using ICSI. One study reported a 13% pregnancy rate with this approach.

If PCOS persists following pregnancy, hormone therapy or surgery may be recommended to offset the long-term risk of developing either diabetes or a heart condition. In women under 35, using birth control pills is the simplest solution to regulating ovarian function.

See: Prolactinemia, Fertility drugs, IVF

62. PREMATURE OVARIAN FAILURE (PREMENOPAUSE): *How can I find out if premenopause is happening to me? One of my friends is barely 35 years old, yet her doctor has diagnosed her as perimenopausal. I thought change of life didn't happen until a woman was at least over 45. Can there be some mistake?*

When it comes to subjects that are taboo, menopause is right up there with death. They may be facts of life, but most of us would rather not discuss them. Luckily, the issue of menopause will precede death for most of us. On the time line of ovarian function, menopause represents the end of menstruation. For the average

American woman, the ovaries stop releasing eggs at the age of 51.

For about six or seven years prior to her very last period, a woman is considered in perimenopause—nearing the climacteric—as female hormone production slowly shuts down. Your friend will probably face menopause in her early forties. With a reduction in estrogen production, ovulation becomes less predictable. Symptoms of this hormonal change may include hot flashes, mood swings, and dryness in the skin and vagina.

When estrogen production slows down in a woman under 40, her diagnosis is premature ovarian failure. This is an irreversible condition for which there is no treatment. Why does this happen? Most common reasons include pelvic infection, endometriosis, or congenital defects. Ovarian tissue is vulnerable to attack by acute inflammation or a chronic condition such as endometriosis. Some women are born with ovaries that don't produce eggs (Turner's syndrome). But if your doctor considers you a good candidate, the donor egg route is a viable option to parenthood.

63. THYROID PROBLEMS (HYPOTHYROIDISM): *Can a thyroid condition be creating a fertility problem for me? I have heard of treatments, including heparin therapy and even blood transfusions, that can correct this situation. Is there any hope for us?*

Your thyroid glands, which are located on either side of your neck along the trachea, regulate proper growth and metabolism in the body. Where reproduction is concerned, they ensure the production of hormones that control ovulation. Where the level of thyroid-stimulating hormone (TSH) is high, you may not be ovulating regularly and may exhibit high prolactin levels (prolactin is the hormone that signals milk production). Where your level is low, synthetic hormone therapy can restore the balance.

How do you know if your thyroid is creating a fertility problem? If you find yourself complaining about chronic fatigue, this might be your first clue. You may have a weight problem, an irregular cycle, or a high level of prolactin. Protruding eyeballs may be another symptom. During my workup one of the doctors at the practice looked at the shape of my eyes and suspected a possible thyroid disorder. A blood test will reveal whether your thyroid is underactive. (Nothing showed up in my case.)

Antithyroid antibodies are now suspect as undermining the success of IVF. Although women with these antibodies are likely to develop underactive thyroids, the risk of miscarriage is not universal. Usually thyroid problems can be successfully controlled through medication. A controversial therapy based on monthly immunoglobulin injections has been introduced in recent years to reduce antibody levels. The notion is that intravenous immunoglobulin (IVIG) injections will protect the fetus from glitches in the immune system. As of this writing, only a handful of doctors are offering this controversial service.

See: Autoimmune dysfunction (Antiphospholipid antibodies)

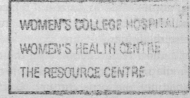

64. UNEXPLAINED INFERTILITY (IDIOPATHIC):
How can fertility drugs help couples like us who have
been diagnosed with unexplained infertility? Why
should I subject my body to fertility drugs when it's
possible we can conceive naturally? We both are 35
years old. Even though we are relieved that neither of
us is responsible for our lack of success, now we don't
know which course of action to follow. . . . Now that
I have been diagnosed with unexplained infertility, I
feel foolish about the careful way I used birth control
over the past five years. In retrospect, it seems like such
a waste of time and energy. I'm upset that my body has
played such a cruel trick on me. My anger sometimes
overwhelms me. Is this a typical reaction?

The medical field of fertility is so young that not all
the causes have yet been identified. When diagnosing a
couple, the specialist measures six factors, beginning
with a semen analysis. The five remaining factors are all
measures of the woman's reproductive health: tubal,
ovulatory, cervical, uterine, and peritoneal. If the results of all these tests come back normal, the diagnosis—for lack of a better one—becomes "unexplained
infertility."

As of this writing, one in 10 of all reported fertility
cases falls into this frustrating category. (For those with
a diagnosis, reasons are divided about equally between
male and female factor.) If this is your diagnosis, you
may be dealing with mixed emotions. How do you fix
something that isn't broken? Any ambivalence is further complicated by a natural reluctance to treat an undiagnosed condition, which may be an expensive
exercise besides.

Medical researchers are on the case, trying to identify the factors for the unexplained population. When
age is not the issue, further tests may uncover more

subtle chemical imbalances or immunological responses. The focus is on creating good-quality embryos and improving the odds of implantation. Often your RE may recommend a course of action appropriate to your age and medical history.

For the patient, medical intervention may help you feel that you're taking action. Commonly, several cycles of intrauterine insemination (IUI) may follow the unexplained diagnosis since this is a fairly noninvasive and affordable route. If undiagnosed antibodies are present in the mucus, IUI will help. Sometimes a normally innocuous organism in the mucus, called ureaplasma, may interfere with fertilization. When both cervical mucus and semen test positive for this organism, antibiotic therapy may come under discussion. Doxycycline seems to cure this condition in one out of two cases. As a rule of thumb, assess the direction of your treatment after three cycles of any one procedure if no progress is made.

Feelings of anger and frustration with this diagnosis are natural following so many invasive medical procedures. Try not to take it out on yourself or your partner. Instead reach out for support whether from a counselor or from a Resolve volunteer. Sometimes taking a vacation from treatment will give you the perspective you need on this detour from your life's blueprint.

65. UTERUS ANOMALY—Insufficient or Double/ T-shaped: According to my gynecologist, my uterus is (one of the above), which reduces my chances of carrying a pregnancy. Is there anything that can be done to correct the situation? . . . TIPPED UTERUS: Since my uterus is tilted, will I have trouble getting pregnant? That's what I've always heard.

If you were born with a tipped uterus, the angle of your uterus has no bearing at all on the ability to conceive, according to the latest research. While the proper position for the uterus is leaning against the bladder, about one in five women is born with a uterus that leans back toward the rectum. In order to be a problem, it would have to be tilted as a result of pelvic adhesions. In the past doctors tightened uterine ligaments in a routine operation to correct the angle. But unless you are in discomfort, you can rule out this congenital anomaly as a reason for infertility.

If the angle of your uterus changed in recent years due to the sudden appearance of adhesions, that's a different story. In that case your diagnosis will probably be peritoneal factor infertility. Common causes for this syndrome include PID and endometriosis. Or the shift in angle may follow childbirth since the uterine ligaments may stretch and become weakened. Chronic backache and constipation are symptoms of this syndrome. Depending on the severity of symptoms, your doctor may recommend inserting a piece of plastic (pessary) to adjust the uterine angle, not to correct a fertility problem. Surgery is the option of last resort.

PART IV

TREATMENTS

CONVENTIONAL
MEDICAL METHODS

66. ANTIBIOTIC THERAPY: I have heard of couples trying to get pregnant for years who got pregnant quickly after going on antibiotics. Which test shows an infection in either partner?

While experts do not agree on the degree to which vaginal infections may compromise fertility, they do acknowledge that excess discharge may depress sperm motility. Since vaginitis may be asymptomatic, it is a good idea to get a Pap smear to determine whether there are unwanted bacteria lurking in the cervix. Men may carry the same bacteria, so it's advisable that your partner consult a urologist for a diagnosis as well.

Current fertility research has identified a new possible culprit that is associated with vaginitis—namely, mycoplasma. These hostile microorganisms found in the cervix are being studied to determine whether they interact with bacteria to prevent sperm from entering the uterus. A standard prescription for tetracycline may clear this situation up in 10 days. I know of one couple who enjoyed immediate benefits from this therapy and successfully conceived two children after years of fruitless trying.

Remember, one possible side effect of antibiotic therapy is yeast infection, so women may need to take preventive measures like eating yogurt or using antiyeast medication.

67. ASSISTED HATCHING (MICROMANIPULA-TION OF EMBRYO TO ENHANCE IMPLANTA-TION): After Pergonal therapy my doctor found that my embryos were not maturing at a proper rate. How will assisted hatching affect the outcome?

A little coaxing in the lab may help improve the odds of implantation for a good embryo, especially for the patient over 39. Natural hatching is the process that follows once an embryo reaches the uterus. When the zona pellucida (the membrane that contains the embryo) opens and the embryo attaches itself to the endometrium so they adhere like two pieces of Velcro, it has "hatched." For the older couple in IVF treatment who have produced good-quality embryos without a pregnancy the hope is that implantation will be enhanced following mechanical hatching.

In order to weaken the thick zona more commonly associated with older women, a chemical may be applied to the embryos prior to transfer in order to facilitate hatching. The procedure takes place once the embryos have passed the eight-cell phase, which is about 72 hours—three full days—after fertilization. Embryo transfer then takes place shortly thereafter. Another technique, known as zona drilling, requires the embryologist actually to make a hole in the embryo and strip away the layers with an acid solution (Tyrode's). Protease digestions (PROD), the newest technique, employs an enzyme to strip away the zona. Obviously, the skill and judgment of the technician are crucial to the ultimate success of this delicate process.

Whether assisted hatching exerts any influence upon successful implantation was questioned at a recent

ASRM convention. Results of a small study at the Jones Institute in Virginia indicated no improvement in implantation or pregnancy rates following this procedure. Further research will determine the feasibility of offering this option in the future.

68. CO-CULTURE: *I've heard that this technique works for people who have "failed" standard IVF treatment. Is it true that embryos thrive in this medium and enhance success rates?*

Perhaps the most discouraging aspect of IVF is having a cycle canceled following fertility drug therapy because of a lack of good-quality embryos for transfer. Placing good-quality eggs and sperm together in a traditional IVF culture medium does not always ensure viable embryos.

In the mid-1990s a team of embryologists made a radical discovery that encouraged the development of good embryos. Adding cells from the fallopian tubes of cows into the IVF medium to create a "co-culture" medium helped reverse poor embryo quality for one third of couples who had faced this problem. What is the secret ingredient? Not even Dr. Klaus Wiemer of Presbyterian Hospital, Charlotte, North Carolina, who developed this technique, knows for sure except to observe that it has a beneficial effect. Further research has found that the addition of a woman's endometrial tissue to the medium may have the same positive influence on embryo development as the cow tissue. While this is good news for embryo development, pregnancy is still contingent upon successful implantation.

As with most fertility therapy, co-culture works best for women under age 38 when fragmentation is strictly a structural issue. In other words, all 46 chromosomes are in place but weakness exists in the egg's cell wall or skeleton. When fragmentation is symptomatic of chromosomal abnormality (aneuploidy), as is more common among women over 40, it signals a birth defect.

One of the pioneers in the co-culture field, the St. Barnabas program in the New York metropolitan area, claims embryo improvement in about three out of four patients under 40 and one out of two over 40. And this new technology comes with the relatively reasonable incremental price tag of $500.

Despite the encouraging developments with this technique, it may be too early to measure its benefits. Research is still scant on the subject, and statistics are not yet available. While embryo quality may improve with co-culture, skeptics question the ultimate success rates. The question remains: Is the co-culture the secret ingredient to a successful cycle or would it have been a good cycle anyway? The issue of cow tissue is also sparking debate. Some experts have reservations about what kind of long-term effect exposing human embryos to cow tissue might have. For the patient facing the question of choosing this therapy, you are committing yourself to fertility research that may become part of routine treatment in the near future.

69. DONOR EGG: I am 44 and my doctor puts my chances of success with my own eggs and IVF at under 5%. The success rate goes up to above 30% if I use donor eggs from a woman under 35. There is no one in my immediate family who can provide eggs. Where do I find a donor?

For a woman with a working uterus but unreliable egg quality, the best opportunity for a full-term, healthy pregnancy is through the donor egg technique. Current national statistics show the take-home-baby rate at about 30% with this technique, with some programs citing one in two.

Essentially, this is IVF treatment with three parties: the couple and a woman with productive ovaries. The donor may be someone you know, a family member, or an anonymous woman whose physical profile closely resembles yours. Studies show that the donor is usually an altruistic young woman with a strong motivation to help an older couple. The standard fee for this service ranges between $2,000 and $3,000 in addition to the IVF cost.

Both the male and female partners submit to thorough physical checkups prior to the designated cycle. As with standard IVF treatment, the donor undergoes controlled superovulation through drug therapy in order to produce a sizable harvest of eggs. Meanwhile the donee begins female hormone therapy (estradiol and progesterone) to prepare her endometrium and put her body in sync with that of the donor so that she will be ready to receive the embryos. Each woman is closely monitored with a series of blood tests.

Following fertility drug therapy, the donor's eggs are retrieved and placed in a petri dish with sperm from the recipient's partner. From that point on the donor's role ends and standard IVF procedure picks up for the couple. Several days after fertilization three or four embryos are transferred into the recipient's uterus in an ambulatory procedure. Excess embryos—should you be fortunate enough to have any—are frozen and stored for future use. The donee continues on a regimen of estradiol and progesterone until her pregnancy test results are analyzed, about two weeks later. If she is pregnant, progesterone therapy extends during the first trimester.

Fertility practices are encouraging women over 40 to

consider seriously the donor egg as the avenue with the best prognosis. If the Day 3 blood test shows high FSH in more than one cycle, the implication is that ovarian function is on the wane. Younger women who have lost their ovaries for a variety of reasons (endometriosis, cancer, or birth defect), or who are facing premature ovarian failure, may benefit from this treatment as well. Although this therapy has been available since 1984, it requires careful reflection to attempt a pregnancy using another woman's genetic material. For the woman whose desire to carry a baby to term outweighs the desire for a biologically related child, this may be a happy solution.

When you look for a suitable donor, your first impulse may be to turn to your family. For women diagnosed with premature ovarian failure (POF), however, this may not be a good option because this syndrome runs in families. According to a recent study at Mount Sinai Hospital in New York City, the rate of canceled cycles ran five times greater with sisters of POF patients than that of cycles using the eggs of anonymous donors. Where there are no genetic considerations, however, sisters are generally the known donors of choice.

Your IVF program will offer other sources if you need an egg donor. Sometimes women in treatment who produce a surfeit may contribute a portion of eggs to the program in exchange for a discount. Since the donee's age is no longer an issue in this scenario, the time pressure does not bear down as heavily. You may have to prepare yourself for some additional waiting since locating a good match is another lengthy process.

Legal issues will concern you, naturally, and should be addressed at the outset. As a rule, all parties are required to consent in writing and agree that the donor's role ends with the egg retrieval. But since each state rules independently on this issue, ask your practitioner to refer you to a local attorney who can answer any questions you have before you embark on treatment.

70. DONOR SPERM: *Can you recommend sperm banks?* . . . *KNOWN DONOR: My brother-in-law is willing to donate his sperm. What are the legal implications? I have some mixed feelings myself.*

Ever since the HIV epidemic, procedures for the donation of bodily secretions have become more stringent, and sperm is no exception. Frozen sperm is now the norm in fertility treatment in order to build in time to check and double-check it.

As recently as 15 years ago sperm banks were accepting donations from male students on the basis of cursory physical histories. Depending upon the demand, the fresh sample might have been immediately put to use in a waiting insemination patient. Nowadays the semen sample is frozen, analyzed, and thoroughly checked over at least three months in order to rule out HIV. According to the American Society for Reproductive Medicine (ASRM), six months is the optimal amount of freezing time prior to insemination in order to allow the sample to be ready for the AIDS antibody blood test and the donor to be retested for HIV. As of this writing, no known cases of HIV have since been connected to insemination. Although the freezing and testing take its toll on the sample, sufficient numbers of sperm are able to make it through the thawing process.

Sperm banks require donors to be under the age of 40. Preference is granted those men who are fathers or have established fertility. In addition to HIV, the sperm bank will screen for hepatitis (B and C), Rh factor, and sexually transmitted diseases. The donor signs an informed consent agreement, and provides a health history. In order to prevent the future possibility of sibling intermarriage, the unwritten rule is a maximum of 10 pregnancies per donor. For a list of sperm banks in your area, contact the ASRM.

As with the donor egg routine, the sperm bank tries to match physical traits of the donor with yours. Even if you decide to use a known donor, the procedure should follow the same protocol with freezing and retesting for HIV. Before you accept an offer of donor sperm, it is advisable to consult a lawyer about your state's definition of paternity in order to avoid future complications. Once the sperm is deemed clean and healthy, the donee can be inseminated during an office appointment on her day of ovulation. A speculum is inserted into the vagina, and the washed sperm may be injected directly into the uterus (IUI), a procedure that shows better success than intravaginal insemination (IVI). Although the process takes five minutes, you can expect to spend anywhere from 10 minutes or more resting on the examination table depending upon your doctor's judgment.

How successful is donor sperm? While the key to success is contingent upon the age and reproductive health of the woman, the fact that sperm must be frozen and thawed takes its toll on the sample. Current statistics report a range of 8 to 15% success per cycle. While donor sperm is an excellent source for the single woman, the ICSI revolution may eclipse this option for the couple with male factor.

71. EMBRYO DEVELOPMENT (Preimplantation Genetic Diagnosis) Part a) BIOPSY: I have frozen embryos in storage at my clinic. I'm considering a transfer but would like some information about the embryos. What will an embryo biopsy show? Is it a replacement for amniocentesis? What happens if we discover they're all defective?

Genetic testing is nerve-racking for any pregnant woman, but especially for one who conceives after fertility treatment. I summarily refused to undergo the chorionic villi sample (CVS) test in the first trimester after hearing rumors that it increased the risk of miscarriage and, worse, was known to snip fingers and toes off the fetus. Next I grappled with the inevitable amniocentesis, which is part of the pregnancy process after age 35, and takes place at the end of the first trimester just when you thought you were home free. While amnio is a voluntary test, terminating at four months because of genetic abnormality can be a devastating decision. Emotionally how much easier it would be to make the decision prior to conception.

While it is not widely available, embryologists have developed a procedure known as preimplantation genetic diagnosis (PGD) as part of the boutique of fertility services. At this time it is not a standard part of treatment. Selected IVF programs use this technique on the embryos of patients who are known carriers of genetic defects (Down syndrome, cystic fibrosis, etc.). For the average patient over age 35 amnio is still the final hurdle you must cross along your path to biological parenthood.

A brand-new diagnosis emerged in 1996 thanks to the development of PGD: chromosomal translocation. About one in 100 couples in fertility treatment have presented with this genetic abnormality: 10 times the average. Problems occur when two different chromosomes interchange pieces and enhance the risk of congenital malformations. PGD screening tests include one for the egg, if the woman is the known carrier, and another for the embryo when the man is the carrier.

For the egg, the test is scheduled immediately following retrieval. At ovulation the egg produces a pair of short-lived small cells (polar bodies) that degenerate quickly in the natural sequence of events. For testing purposes, if removed within six hours after egg retrieval, they offer a clear chromosomal picture of the embryo. Normal cells are comprised of 23 chromosomes each. Through gentle aspiration the polar body is removed from beneath the shell (zona pellucida) and the egg is returned to the incubator for fertilization. Using a new process called FISH (fluorescence in situ hybridization), or chromosome painting, color probes identify any imbalance in the polar body. Results are analyzed, and a decision can be made prior to transfer.

Since sperm do not have polar bodies, analysis must focus on the embryonic cells. One or two cells (blastomeres) are analyzed using the FISH technique. Instead of analyzing the chromosomes, the embryologist develops chemical probes to investigate the regions where a translocation is suspected.

Is this procedure harmful to the embryo? It may be too early to determine with assurance, but results show the success rate following PGD to be comparable to success rate without. With so many micromanipulation procedures performed by drilling into the zona pellucida (i.e., ICSI and assisted hatching), experience shows that the egg can withstand such tampering. The embryo recovers its normal development as well. On the downside, some experts believe the integrity of the embryos are compromised following biopsy. Furthermore, PGD may yield faulty results in 10% of the cases, which could mean rejecting healthy embryos. Since for this group of patients healthy eggs may be in short supply, that could limit the success of conceiving with their own eggs.

As of this writing, PGD is offered in the New York metropolitan area at St. Barnabas and New York/Cornell, in Chicago at Illinois Masonic, in Houston at Baylor, and in Fairfax, Virginia, at the Genetics and IVF Institute.

Part b) EMBRYO RANKING: Are the odds of success better with better-quality embryos? How are they graded?

Embryos are graded according to overall appearance and the rate of cell division on a scale of one (top) to four. Good embryos need good eggs and proper culture medium in the lab to ensure timely development. Characteristics of a "good-looking" embryo are a consistent color (like straw), a lack of blemishes (spots or speckles), a healthy texture, and a minimum of fragmentation. High levels of fragmentation are associated with chromosomal abnormalities and are more common in embryos of older women.

As the embryo develops prior to implantation, cells will divide more than once into smaller halves. As long as the division continues to occur in pairs (from two to four, etc.), the outlook is good. The initial cell division takes place about 36 hours after fertilization and then accelerates to every 12 hours. By the time of transfer on the second day after retrieval the embryo should have reached the two- to four-cell stage. According to this schedule, by the third day the embryo is in the eight- to 16-cell stage. Embryos that conform to this time frame will receive a high grade. The culture medium is key to keeping embryo development on track.

As long as the uterine lining is receptive and no autoimmune factors apply, yes, better-quality embryos (grade 1 or 1.5) are more likely to implant. They are also more likely to result in a multiple pregnancy. According to recent statistics at the NYU Medical Center, 60% of the pregnancies in its under 40-year-old patients are multiple. With three embryos transferred in the under 35 group, and four in the 35 to 39, multiples developed when two or more embryos ranked 1.5 or better.

Keep in mind, however, that lower-grade embryos may implant and become viable pregnancies as well. It's simply that a crop of TQE is a more reliable predictor of a positive outcome as well as a measure of multiples. One specialist told me that future success is implied if a patient produces 12 or more embryos in a single cycle.

Part c) EMBRYO TRANSFER: What is the standard number of embryos that are transferred into the uterus in the IVF process?

While there are legal parameters in other countries (three embryos in the United Kingdom and Canada, two in Australia), no fixed number of embryos is attached in an IVF transfer in the United States. By tacit agreement three are ideal, with four the maximum transferred per cycle in order to contain the possibility of a multiple gestation. However, depending upon the age of the patient and the embryo grade, the doctor may recommend transferring more. (In an unsuccessful cycle I had seven low-ranked embryos transferred.)

Since every case is handled individually on the basis of the fertility profile of the two partners, the number of embryos transferred is a judgment call based on the knowledge and experience of the reproductive endocrinologist. Although no federal government regulations are in place, the field is self-regulated through the American Society of Reproductive Medicine (ASRM) as well as state-issued licenses that cover each aspect of treatment from blood tests to storage of sperm or embryos. Through the ASRM, standards are evolving, although it remains to be seen whether they will be legally binding. Some states, such as New York, are exploring whether their departments of health should set fixed guidelines for IVF practitioners. Meanwhile, the Wyden bill is attempting to establish some parameters in the field.

If the United States follows the trend of the United Kingdom in limiting the number of embryos per transfer to a maximum of three, this may spur more research in the area of preimplantation cytogenetics in order to build up success rates.

72. FERTILITY DRUGS Part a) PILL: Isn't there a fertility pill? How does it work?

The fertility pill (brand name Clomid) is composed of the drug clomiphene citrate, a form of antiestrogen similar to tamoxifen, a medication for breast cancer prevention. "Fertility pill" is a misnomer because it is specifically indicated for women with either ovulation issues or a luteal phase defect, or about four in 10 infertile women. Ironically, it was originally going to be marketed as a form of oral contraception designed to suppress female hormones. Instead its effect may trigger each ovary to release an egg during a single cycle, raising the stakes of conceiving twins up to 10%. (Fewer than 1% conceive triplets on this medication.)

Where blocked tubes are not an issue, clomiphene therapy may raise your odds close to those of fertile couples. The ASRM reports that after six cycles Clomid yields 50% success and 80% after 12 cycles. Usually the prescription begins at Day 3 of your menstrual cycle and lasts five days. For the first cycle the daily dose begins at 50 milligrams. Depending on how your body responds, the dosage in subsequent cycles may be increased to three times that strength in order to stimulate response.

The drug tricks the brain into increasing the secretion of follicle-stimulating hormone (FSH) and luteinizing hormone (LH) into the bloodstream by blocking the estrogen receptors in the hypothalamus. To compensate for what the body perceives as an estrogen deficiency, the pituitary gland then pumps out excess female hormones, which should help cultivate a mature follicle or two in the first half of the cycle. Ovulation—the release of an egg by the follicle—follows about a week after the prescription has ended.

In cases where your body doesn't respond to Clomid the doctor may add an injection of human chorionic gonadotropin (hCG) to your protocol. This derivative from the urine of pregnant women triggers the release of the egg from the dominant follicle. Close monitoring through ultrasound and blood tests follow the follicle's development prior to the administering of hCG.

If Clomid does not help your case, your doctor will move on to a different therapy. General consensus is a maximum of 12 cycles of Clomid. Since Clomid is inexpensive (about $20 per cycle), the temptation is to try it no matter what your diagnosis. I fell into this trap and convinced my doctor to prescribe Clomid for eight cycles until I developed strange headaches. To be fair, at the time my diagnosis was still "unexplained." Although I was satisfying my urge to be proactive about getting pregnant, I was also delaying the appropriate treatment.

Part b) HUMAN MENOPAUSAL GONADO-TROPIN—Superovulation: My doctor has prescribed Pergonal, and my husband will administer the injections. What's in Pergonal? Why is it so expensive? . . . I've heard that there is a new form of hMG that is easier to inject than Pergonal. Is this true? . . .

EXCESS: What do I do with leftover fertility drugs now that I'm expecting?

Driving the field of assisted reproductive technology—as well as the headlines of multiple births—is the potent fertility drug commercially known as Pergonal. (Alternately, the other brand name is Humegon.) An estimated one in five Pergonal-induced pregnancies result in multiples, with twins predominating. As in most cases of multiple gestation, the risk of giving birth prematurely increases with the number of fetuses.

Human menopausal gonadotropin (hMG, brand name, Pergonal) is composed of the two pituitary hormones that control ovulation, follicle-stimulating hormone (FSH) and luteinizing hormone (LH). Pergonal works directly on the ovaries to enhance the production of mature follicles. Under natural circumstances your body produces one follicle (two at most) and absorbs the undeveloped ones. Pergonal "rescues" those little ones and allows them to mature so that they can potentially fertilize.

This powerful drug is derived from a waste product; it is culled from the urine of postmenopausal women. Religious convents, for one, are good sources for collecting raw material. But because of its limited availability, the cost for a single cycle of a Pergonal prescription now runs about $2,000. Although it can be purchased abroad for less, you will not have the FDA approval that indicates safe use. Secondly, customs may confiscate the drugs upon reentering the U.S.

Once you are introduced to Pergonal therapy, you will be committed to fertility treatment in a way you probably never anticipated. Treatment usually begins around Day 3 and continues for a week or more. First of all, your husband or a family member will be recruited to give you the daily injections of one or two ampules. A short demonstration in the doctor's office is required prior to the beginning of treatment, and you will receive careful training in the proper way to administer the drug. To date, I have never heard of any cases of complications arising from this aspect of the treatment.

The Pergonal injection is given intramuscularly, usually in the upper outer part of the buttock. You should alternate hips during the course of the prescription. I have met women who were able to self-administer the injections, but they are the exceptions. At the other end of the spectrum I have spoken to those who needed to hire a nurse for a small fee. Directly following the retraction of the needle apply a hot compress to the site. (A washcloth will do.) The heat will dissipate the medication through the bloodstream and soothe the injection site. Incorporate the washcloth into the routine, and you will avoid developing a sore hip.

Close monitoring of ovarian response means you will check in at the doctor's office daily for ultrasound and blood tests to track estrogen levels. Timing is crucial. You need to take the medication at the same time of day during the course of the prescription. Always check the expiration date on the ampules when preparing the injection.

As soon as one or two follicles have reached maturity (about 20 millimeters), a final injection of human chorionic gonadotropin (hCG) will trigger ovulation. Depending on dosage and response, you may produce anywhere from a few to two dozen (or more) viable follicles. If the doctor is concerned about ovarian hyperstimulation, he or she may forgo the hCG shot, and that means the cycle is canceled. Signs of hyperstimulation begin with enlargement of the ovaries from their usual almond size and may lead to "weeping," in which fluid collects in the abdomen.

If you should choose to obtain fertility drugs abroad, inform your doctor so that the medications can be examined prior to injection. Obviously, you should check the packaging and expiration dates before purchasing.

As for unused vials, ask your program if you can donate unopened medications to it directly for redistribution.

Part c) FOLLICLE-STIMULATING HORMONE (FSH): I'm on a combination of Metrodin and Pergonal. How do they interact?

Metrodin is simply the brand name for follicle-stimulating hormone (FSH), a product of the pituitary gland. It's a diluted form of Pergonal, with only a slight amount of luteinizing hormone (LH). FSH works directly on the ovaries to enhance follicle development. It's most often prescribed for women who have low or normal FSH and high LH levels, such as those with polycystic ovarian syndrome. It may also be combined with Pergonal treatment when extra stimulation is required to elicit good response from the ovaries. For example, both drugs may be indicated for IVF treatment in order to yield a good harvest of eggs. The odds of conceiving a multiple pregnancy with this medication is comparable to Pergonal treatment, about 20%.

Just like Pergonal, Metrodin is derived from the urine of postmenopausal women and is injected intramuscularly into the hip for about seven days. Always apply a hot compress to the site after each injection to minimize residual soreness. Blood levels need to be closely followed, and the growth of the follicles needs to be measured daily with ultrasound.

As of late 1996, Fertinex, a more purified form of FSH, received FDA approval after gaining widespread acceptance abroad. This new fertility drug soon may alter the basic ART protocol to stimulate superovulation. Most appealing about Fertinex is the fact that it is administered subcutaneously, which makes it easier to inject yourself. As with Pergonal, Fertinex therapy begins on Day 2 or 3 and continues for about 10 days. Studies show it to be equally effective as the intramuscular version. Will Fertinex help to lower the high probability of multiple births? It certainly is the hope within the industry.

Part d) LUPRON (Gonadotropin-Releasing Hormone antagonist): *Lupron is part of my protocol. Why isn't it FDA-approved? Should I worry?*

Lupron is the synthetic form of gonadotropin-releasing hormone (GnRH), which controls the secretion of FSH and LH by the pituitary. By suspending LH production, Lupron puts a stop to the process of ovulation and offers Pergonal treatment better control over follicle stimulation. "Down regulation" of these hormones removes the selection of a dominant follicle that occurs on a monthly basis. Instead many follicles may reach maturity in response to Pergonal therapy; in theory this could translate into more embryos. Since female hormonal activity is suspended, your body is in an artificial state of menopause. Consequently, you may have a little preview of side effects from hot flashes to mood swings. (I did not experience any extreme symptoms.) A nurse at my program called Lupron the conductor in the orchestra of drugs that precede IVF.

Unlike Pergonal and Metrodin, Lupron injections are subdermal and can be self-administered. The needle is small, similar to a darning needle, and can be inserted without any discomfort. Lupron therapy begins at the end of your cycle (about Day 24) and goes on for between two and three weeks. Of course, your doctor's office will give you full instructions before the beginning of the prescription. I clearly recall scoffing at the Lupron training session at the notion that I would actually inject myself! Minutes later I was amazed when I allowed the little needle to puncture the surface of my thigh without getting squeamish. Crossing each hurdle of the fertility sweepstakes is all part of the process.

Why isn't Lupron FDA-approved for fertility treatment? This drug is mainly prescribed for prostate cancer and has been approved for that protocol. While it has become a part of standard IVF therapy, funds are simply not available to underwrite a major study at this time to gain final approval for this aspect of fertility treatment.

Part e) PROGESTERONE: This is the most uncomfortable injection of all. Can you explain?

This hormone is aptly named to reflect its function in the beginning of pregnancy: *pro* (for) + *ges* (tation) + *terone* (the hormonal suffix). Following ovulation, your body releases it to help build uterine lining for secure embryo implantation. When you're on an ART protocol, progesterone is prescribed to maximize the receptivity of your endometrium.

Unfortunately, progesterone is oily by nature and requires a bigger needle than Pergonal. Since it takes a while to seep into the bloodstream, the injection may feel prolonged. Again, as with all injections, a warm compress can help alleviate subsequent swelling at the site. After trying progesterone suppositories, I insisted on using them instead. The drawback is the possibility that the drug will leak out of the body rather than be absorbed by it. Some women find it messy and resent wearing a sanitary pad. Although most fertility practitioners insist on injections, you do have two alternatives. (Progesterone exists in tablet form as well.) It's worth discussing with your RE.

73. FROZEN EMBRYOS (Cryopreservation): I've heard that IVF success rates are better with the transfer of frozen embryos during a natural cycle. Should I opt to freeze all my embryos for better results? Can I freeze my eggs?

After taking the fertility drug cocktail required prior to egg retrieval, I wondered how any woman could get pregnant feeling as crampy and medicated as I did. With all those drugs in my bloodstream, I was skeptical that one embryo could implant properly. After all, if a simple bottle of beer warns pregnant women of the evil effects of alcohol on the unborn, conventional wisdom would follow that drugs—prescription or otherwise— may have a harmful effect.

While I have met many women who conceived on the first transfer, it seemed like a long shot to me. On the other hand, returning for a transfer once my body returned to normal made sense. Both times that I got pregnant with IVF it was with frozen embryos. Of course, success is contingent upon two factors: a program that can accommodate frozen embryos and, most important, their proper thawing.

If you produce a sufficient number of good-quality embryos that can withstand the freezing process, it may work in your favor. Experts have confirmed that my hunch was right: Endometrial receptivity may be superior during a frozen cycle. Another incremental benefit is the higher rate of singleton pregnancies with this technique. Yet SART Report results show success with frozen embryos hovering at 16% per transfer, 5% below IVF rates. In 1996 6,900 transfers of cryopreserved embryos yielded 1,100 deliveries.

Does it make sense to freeze all your embryos for transfer at a later date? Your decision depends on the number of good-quality embryos available and the thawing success rate at your clinic. Actually, thawing rates are encouraging, according to the 1996 SART Report, which cites 96% of the cases progressed to transfer. Certainly it is an avenue worth exploring and discussing with your doctor.

While cryopreservation works for both sperm and embryos, as of this writing eggs are too delicate to be stored this way. But things may change quickly; at least one pregnancy has recently been reported using a frozen egg. Until eggs can be preserved safely, however, banking your embryos is a worthwhile effort. A single cycle with a good egg harvest and a high level of fertilization can result in two take-home babies.

74. GAMETE INTRAFALLOPIAN TRANSFER (GIFT): *I've heard that success rates with GIFT are better for women over 40. Since I'm 42 this information could be crucial to my treatment. Is it true?*

What a nice ring the acronym GIFT has to it. After undergoing the rigors of the workup and the fertility medications, a gift at the end of the road would be welcome. In fact, the doctor who introduced this technique, Dr. Ricardo Asch, deliberately tried to convey the notion of the gift of life. This particular GIFT is a combination of *gametes* (sperm plus egg) transferred *intra* the *fallopian tubes*. Fertilization is expected to take place in the woman's body, not in a laboratory as with in vitro. If an embryo develops, with luck, it will implant in the uterus.

Who can benefit from GIFT? Patients who have good fallopian tubes yet have reason to believe that there are mitigating factors keeping egg and sperm apart. Good candidates include those with diagnoses of mild endometriosis, immunological factors (antibodies), cervical problems, or cases of unexplained infertility.

The GIFT procedure begins with fertility drug therapy to stimulate the production of mature follicles. Once the follicles are ready, a laparoscopy is scheduled in the operating room *usually* under general anesthesia. In the first part of the procedure the eggs are retrieved with a laparoscope via a belly button incision. The surgeon examines the eggs, grades them for maturity (one through four), and selects some to be combined in a petri dish with the sperm, which has been specially washed. Shortly after, the mixture is transferred via catheter to one or both fallopian tubes. Success rates are encouraging at 28% per retrieval. To contain the possibility of a multiple pregnancy, most practitioners limit the number of eggs transferred to two. Any embryos that may result from the retrieval may be frozen and stored for potential in vitro transfer at a later date.

Is the older woman more apt to find success with GIFT? No, there is no known technique to reverse the effects of age. Today's research shows donor egg in tandem with IVF yields the best success for this age group. Originally it was believed that since IVF results are so abysmal for the over 40 population, GIFT would offer a better opportunity. After all, this procedure ensures the rendezvous of egg with sperm at the right place and the right time. But subsequent studies have refuted the notion that these factors can offset age, and the take-home-baby rates seem comparable to IVF.

75. GESTATIONAL HOST (surrogate): My RE says my uterus won't carry a baby to term. What options are open to me? How do I find a carrier?

For women with good ovarian function but a non-working (or absent) uterus, biological parenthood is possible through the use of another woman's uterus (gestational host). Essentially, the host acts as an incubator for an embryo produced by the couple.

The diagnosis of a nonfunctioning uterus forces you to turn to outside sources. Like patients in search of donor eggs, you require the services of a more fertile woman. Psychologically this issue may have widespread repercussions that can be addressed in counseling.

As in the case of any donor, you may turn to your family first. Stories of grandmothers carrying babies for their daughters or sisters helping sisters have appeared in the national press. Not everyone is comfortable with the long-term implications of using a relative for this purpose. If this is not an option for you, agencies exist to help you locate someone willing to provide this service for a fee. Finding a reliable, healthy host outside the family circle requires careful research, especially since this service is not yet legal in every state. One good resource is The Organization for Parents Through Surrogacy (OPTS), which has national headquarters on the West Coast. Since the process is costly ($50,000 or more for IVF plus maternity) you need to understand all the legal implications.

The 1996 SART Report includes 64 programs that

treated more than 200 cases of host uterus transfer. Of these, about nine in 10 progressed to retrieval, with transfer following in almost every case. No ectopic pregnancies were noted. The overall delivery rate compares to statistics for the under 39 IVF population at one in three, with 27% resulting in twins and 6% in triplets. (No sets of greater multiples were reported.) Also encouraging is the fact that only two of the 67 babies born through this technology exhibited birth defects.

See: Ten Key Fertility Contacts

76. HEPARIN (ANTICOAGULANT) THERAPY: *Why is the medical community split on this issue? What is the controversy surrounding antiphospholipid antibodies?*

Endocrinologists are on the case to find reasons why miscarriage is so prevalent in a large majority of the infertile population. Among the top suspects are glitches in a woman's immune system, such as the counterproductive development of antiphospholipid antibodies. These destructive molecules undermine the reproductive system and mobilize to cut off nourishment to a growing embryo. Research on this subject has been pioneered by Dr. Geoffrey Sher of Pacific Fertility.

Phospholipids are present in every cell of the body. Trouble may begin if antibodies set off a chain of events that make it impossible for the phospholipids to do their job in the placenta and uterus. Viewing the fertilized egg as an invader, the antibodies mobilize to choke off its blood supply. This activity may cause clots to form. Depending upon how much influence they exert, their presence could result in an underweight baby or, more tragically, in a pattern of miscarriage.

While the theory of an antibody malfunction sounds

reasonable as a factor, it is not yet a universally accepted diagnosis by members of the ASRM. Some experts believe that antibodies alone are too simple an explanation and that further studies may uncover other more complex elements at work. Despite the difference of opinion on the cause, there is agreement that heparin is working on some aspect of the reproductive system to correct infertility. One mid-1990s study has shown that two thirds of women with endometriosis test positive for antibodies, which may shed light on the underlying pathology of that condition.

If you are found to have a high level of antiphospholipid antibodies, the risk of developing a circulatory problem may be heightened. To counteract the antibodies, you have to consider whether you subscribe to the theory that you need to protect the blood supply to the fetus. One fairly harmless antidote is baby aspirin therapy. Your RE may recommend one a day in order to thin your blood and prevent potential clotting that may cut off nourishment to the fetus. Or heparin treatment may be indicated. Standard prescription is one subcutaneous injection self-administered twice a day for the first half of your pregnancy.

77. INSEMINATION (Artificial/Intrauterine): Is this procedure painful? I've heard mixed reports. Is there a limit to the number of inseminations possible? I once met a woman who got lucky after 15 inseminations. Does it help the success rate to combine fertility drugs with insemination? What's the difference between artificial and intrauterine insemination?

When no definitive diagnosis has yet been made and you want to feel proactive, insemination usually comes under discussion. First, your RE must determine if you are a good candidate. Leading factors of infertility have to be ruled out—namely, tubal and ovulation factors for the woman, as well as male factor (unless you're using donor sperm). Obviously the ovaries must be releasing good eggs, the tubes must be clear in order to help the sperm and egg meet, and the sperm must be able to swim effectively. For men whose sperm is marginal, you may elect to go with donor sperm or mix a sample with that of a donor to enhance results.

The procedure is scheduled for the days just before ovulation (Day 10 to 14). Cervical mucus must be translucent and friendly ("fern" pattern). For best results, your RE may test it again at this time. Generally, sperm are delivered fresh in the morning so that they can be washed and prepared. If you bring the sample from home, make sure the container remains warm so that the sperm survive the trip. The procedure takes place on the examination table with the woman's feet in stirrups. Once the speculum is in place, the sperm sample is placed onto the cervix (intracervical, ICI) or directly into the uterus (IUI), which is farther along the reproductive tract than nature would place it. A sponge or cap may be inserted into the vagina to contain the sperm in the body. Depending upon your doctor, you will remain prone for at least 15 minutes or longer. Some specialists recommend two inseminations per cycle to keep live sperm in the reproductive tract for optimal results. The second insemination follows 24 hours after the first.

Yes, some discomfort is associated with IUI, which deposits the sperm deeper into the body. The sample must be carefully washed to remove the prostaglandins in the seminal plasma that could potentially trigger painful uterine contractions. For a diagnosis of cervical factor, IUI is ideal because it completely bypasses the cervix and the attendant hostile microorganisms that have been preventing conception.

Depending on your age and your ovulation history, your RE may discuss the possibility of using fertility drugs in tandem with insemination. By producing multiple eggs each month, you may increase the possibility that one will fertilize. While there is no physical ceiling on the number of inseminations a couple may have, psychologically this process can wear you down. Odds of conceiving with fresh sperm are 15% per attempt, or one in six, comparable to the odds of the old-fashioned way. (With frozen sperm, the average number of attempts before success rises to 10.) A previous pregnancy seems to improve the odds in your favor.

78. IN VITRO FERTILIZATION (IVF) Part a) Success Rates Per Age: What are the odds of our success with IVF if I am under 39? Over 40?

Most current official results, based on activity in 249 clinics during 1994, were published by the Society for Assisted Reproductive Medicine (SART) at the end of 1996. According to the bible of the industry known as the SART Report, the national take-home-baby rate per retrieval—based on a total of nearly 34,000—is 21% or about one in five. GIFT and ZIFT showed better success at 28% and 29% (about one in four), respectively, although the patient population is considerably smaller at 4,200 and 900 respectively. By the end of 1994 more than 6,000 babies were born thanks to ART. Nearly two thirds of these were single births (singletons), with twins accounting for 29%, triplets 7% and higher multiple sets another 0.5%.

Why the lag between year of treatment and reporting year? First of all, analyzing the data couldn't begin until October 1995, nine months after the last embryo transfer of 1994. With so many clinics and patients to track, tabulating and publishing the information required another 12 months. Peat Marwick, the national auditing firm, served as the impartial collection center. Finally, 1994 represents the first application of the SART Database Program that is attempting to set parameters for the industry. Submitting data to SART is now mandatory for all members.

Note that of the 249 clinics, 16 programs exceeded the national average by better than 9% with take-home-baby rates of 30% or more. Certainly, you must examine results closely for the practice in which you are enrolled since some specialties are program specific. After 1994 great strides in IVF lab technology have improved success rates considerably, and we can expect the next SART Report to show better take-home-baby rates nationwide.

SART data are divided into four major categories: women over and under the age of 40, with and without male factor. Subcategories include stimulated and unstimulated cycles, frozen transfers, and donor eggs. Results on ICSI, co-culture, and other subsequently introduced technologies were not yet available but stand to improve statistics in future.

Cancellation rate with IVF occurs in one of nine cases for 39 and under, escalating to one in five for over 40. The leading reason that a cycle is called off? No viable embryos, clinically known as "failure to fertilize." This situation is more apt to occur where a male factor is present. (Again, nowadays ICSI may be able to reverse this trend.) Also on the downside, one in 100 transfers results in an ectopic (tubal) pregnancy, which must be terminated.

National clinical pregnancy rates for the 39 and under group with no male factor are quite encouraging;

nearly one in three IVF cases will have a positive pregnancy test. From a total of 15,000 stimulated (medicated) cycles, nearly 2,000 were canceled. Of the 13,000 remaining cycles, 4,500 pregnancies ensued. Deducting for miscarriage in almost 20% of this group, 1994 recorded 3,700 deliveries. Adding a male factor to the formula depresses the results to one in five. From a sample of 4,500 cases 1,000 pregnancies resulted in 900 babies.

Over age 40 the scenario slips to one pregnancy in eight cases, down to one in 10 with a male factor (predating ICSI). Specifically, in 2,700 cycles 600 were canceled. Since miscarriage escalates to 35%, of the nearly 400 pregnancies in this subset 250 babies were born in 1994.

Another syndrome that may compromise IVF outcome is hydrosalpinx, which occurs when the fimbriae at the end of the fallopian tube become inflamed and create a fluid-filled sac. The secretions that become trapped erode the uterine lining and discourage implantation. In this case some experts are recommending the surgical removal of the tubes to improve the odds of success.

Part b) IVF BIRTH DEFECTS: *What is the likelihood of birth defects with IVF? Is there any correlation with embryo ranking?*

According to the latest research as of the 1996 convention of the American Society of Reproductive Medicine, the incidence of birth defects among IVF offspring compares directly to that of the population at large. Regardless of how you conceived, 2% of newborns will manifest a birth defect. Medical intervention and treatment prior to gestation do not appear to have a negative impact on the resulting pregnancy.

From cycle to cycle, variables within your body change. One month you may produce "top-quality" embryos, while you don't in the next stimulated cycle. One month is no guarantee for the next attempt. You can't make assumptions based on how you responded last time. In fact, more than 70% of early-stage embryos are lost in the IVF process.

What is a top-quality embryo? An embryo exhibiting less than 5% of structural fragmentation on Day 3 following culture (fertilization). The range spans from grade 1 or 1.5 for a TQE down through grade 4. Yet I've spoken with doctors who have seen grade 4 embryos turn into viable pregnancies as well as grade 1's that failed to implant. Can the difference be due to the mode of transfer? Some doctors believe that the type of catheter used may influence the outcome. Three types are used in the embryo transfer process: Wallace, Tom Cat, and Rocket. In straightforward cases where the uterus and cervix conform to normal shapes, the Wallace catheter is used. Success rates are high with this catheter since it is indicated for cases that do not present any unusual difficulty.

Part c) "NATURAL" IVF (No Fertility Drugs): Can I do IVF without fertility drugs?

In this age of organic foods and natural cosmetics, there is a deep-seated resistance to and concern about the medications required in fertility therapy. Clearly, these must be powerful drugs that are creating a generation rife with twins and triplets. There is no question that the addition of drugs plays a pivotal role in maximizing the success rates of each expensive IVF procedure. With only one or two ova released per month under normal circumstances, it would be a costly proposition to return to the hospital every month for IVF treatment. Although the very first IVF baby, Louise Brown, was conceived without drugs, they are now part of the protocol.

Yes, the "natural" IVF cycle is an option on today's fertility menu but only under certain circumstances. Of the 27,000 cycles covered in the 1996 SART Report, fewer than 2% underwent this form of treatment. Even in this select sample success rates are well below those of medicated IVF cycles at a mere 8% (one in 13). Generally an RE recommends this route as a cheaper, albeit less effective alternative. Of 400 "natural" cycles as reported by 62 programs, half were canceled. With only one or two eggs retrieved, fertilization failure can scrap the cycle. Of 22 ensuing pregnancies, 16 take-home babies were born, including two to women over 40.

For the younger patient with time and good health benefits, natural IVF is available. Besides satisfying the health-conscious patient, it puts controls on the burgeoning multiple pregnancies. By retrieving the one dominant follicle as well as some secondary ones, the reproductive endocrinologist endeavors to produce more than one embryo. Research in this area is in progress to develop new methods that would encourage immature ova to develop outside the body rather than grow them internally through hormone therapy.

Could the season influence results? Is there a more fertile time of the year? According to statistics compiled since 1930, evidence indicates that conception is more likely to occur when the temperature is moderate, between 50 and 70 degrees Fahrenheit. North of the equator spring seems most fertile, with autumn second. It's just the reverse south of the border. Light seems to play a role in fertility as well. For women with irregular cycles, sleeping with a 100 watt lamp burning seemed to put the cycle on the 28-day track. One study showed good results with IVF when eggs were retrieved late in the evening, about 11:00 P.M.

79. INTRACYTOPLASMIC SINGLE SPERM INJECTION (ICSI)—Micromanipulation and Round Spermatid Nuclear Injection (ROSNI): My husband's sperm count is really low. I have heard of a new procedure that requires only one potent sperm. How does it work?

Yes, the mid-1990s introduced a revolutionary technique in the field of infertility that can yield a biological child for couples diagnosed with male factor, even severe cases. Thanks to the efforts of embryologist Gianpiero Palermo, M.D. (originally working in Belgium, now affiliated with the New York/Cornell Center for Reproductive Medicine), a new era in reproductive medicine has made sperm quality moot. All you need is one motile sperm. Now the embryologist can aspirate a single sperm and inject it directly into the egg in a process familiarly called ICSI—intracytoplasmic sperm injection—and create a take-home baby in 65% of this population.

Male factor infertility covers the gamut of sperm issues: low count or quality, poor motility or penetration capability, abnormal shape. Micromanipulation technology to compensate for lacking sperm quality has been incorporated into the IVF program for the past decade. The forerunner in the field, partial zona dissection (PZD), was designed to encourage sperm penetration. With the use of a chemical peel or surgical file, the shell of the ovum (zona pellucida) was opened for easier entry by the sperm. However, fertilization is not guaranteed with PZD, and with multiple sperm (polyspermy) entering the egg too often, nonviable embryos resulted. This led to ICSI's direct precursor, subzonal insertion (SUZI), whereby sperm were placed into the space between the zona and the interior of the egg. Again, there were no controls over how many sperm were entering the egg.

By refining the technology to limit entry to a single sperm, ICSI has made donor sperm almost superfluous in the IVF universe. Dr. Palermo and his colleagues found that even immature round sperm may be removed from the testicle of men with zero sperm count to produce viable embryos. (ROSNI technology, whereby undeveloped sperm are aspirated from the epididymis, is being developed for this purpose.) For the female partner, IVF proceeds as usual with superovulation through fertility drugs. After retrieval, the ICSI magic begins. Since the technique is so new and delicate, the embryologist often makes his or her own ICSI tools for the injection. Success hinges on skill combined with a quality needle.

Rather than mix ova and sperm in the petri dish as in the standard method, the embryologist strips the external covering (cumulus) from the ova and assesses it for maturity. Next, the egg must be held in place while the sperm is inserted. For best results, the sperm must be cleansed and slowed down. Just before insertion the sperm's tail is pinched to prevent it from flailing about and potentially damaging the egg. For the injection the egg is placed either in a petri dish or on a glass slide according to personal preference. The actual shot happens in the blink or two of an eye. Fourteen hours later the egg is checked to determine whether fertilization has occurred, and if all goes well, cleavage should take place on the following day.

80. TUBAL PROCEDURES—CATHETERIZATION (Transcervical Cannulation): Now that my tubes have been diagnosed as blocked and nonfunctioning, I'm looking forward to clearing them out through surgery. Since I am ovulating regularly and my husband's sperm is motile and abundant, I can't wait to correct this problem and conceive at home. Is it really that simple? . . . TUBOPLASTY: After I had an ectopic pregnancy, my tubes were closed off. Still, my doctor informs me that there is a slim possibility of another tubal pregnancy. How can that be? . . .

LASER SURGERY: So many internal problems are correctable with laser. Can it be applied to tubal blockage?

Although fallopian tubes are only about 10 centimeters long, successful repair depends upon which part of this tiny span is afflicted. Each tube is comprised of four parts: the fimbria (fringed area), which borders the ovary and connects with the ampullary portion, which leads to the narrow isthmus before the interstitial, which opens into the uterus. The tubal interior is lined with plush cilia that act like the flaps in a car wash as they propel the egg from the ovary to the uterus. If the sperm meets the egg in the fallopian tube and fertilization takes place, the tube secretes nutrients that are essential for embryo development.

Blockage found in the interstitial (proximal) area responds best to repair—provided that the problem is due to a buildup of proteins and not to tissue damage. (Scarring presents other complications.) To clear the tube, the technician combines catheterization, threaded through the reproductive tract, with the uterine X ray known for short as HSG (hysterosalpingogram). By the pumping of fluid through the catheter the blockage is, one hopes, dislodged and function restored. This technique, commonly known as cannulation, shows improvement in four out of 10 cases.

What if tissue damage is responsible for the proximal blockage? If the cause was tubal inflammation—salpingitis isthmica nodosa (SIN)—surgery may work. Damaged tissue is removed, and the tube is reconnected to the uterus (clinically known as resection and reanastomosis). The success of this procedure, estimated also at four in 10, is contingent on the extent of the damage and the skill of your surgeon. Repair of an organ as delicate as the fallopian tube is attempted just once. If repair surgery (tuboplasty) proves ineffective, you are headed to ART. With risk of an ectopic (tubal) pregnancy close to 10% following repair—three times the rate with IVF—residual scarring may end up undermining your best efforts. Sadly, tubal pregnancies must be terminated since they pose a threat to the mother's life.

Is there hope to repair blockage at the distal (fimbriated) end? Only if your diagnosis is a small hydrosalpinx, a fluid-filled sac that closes off entry from the ovary. The HSG will record the size and location of the hydrosalpinx. Its sac forms when the fimbriae fuse together following an inflammation. Over time accumulated fluids erode the quality of the tubal lining and compromise embryo development. Even if surgery corrects the problem, the good news is tempered by the escalated risk of an ectopic pregnancy: 15% to 20%. Again, extensive scarring in the area may trap the embryo in the tube. IVF prognosis for women with this syndrome may be diminished as the result of long-term erosion of the uterine lining. Surgical removal of the tubes may enhance implantation, according to some experts.

Laser is an integral part of the microsurgery movement associated with assisted reproductive technology.

During laparoscopy or hysteroscopy the microsurgeon may resort to laser repair where appropriate, such as to open mildly blocked tubes. Where laser correction may be most beneficial is for severe cases of polycystic ovarian syndrome (PCOS). When the ovaries don't respond to traditional fertility drug therapy, the RE may opt for laser drilling. Through a laparoscope the surgeon punctures the ovarian surface with the laser beam in more than one place. This procedure temporarily triggers ovulation when nothing worked before.

With recent strides in IVF, your RE may advise you to compare success of repair with ART before you elect to reconstruct your tubes. Despite the fact that your insurance may cover reconstruction and especially in the case of distal blockage, repair surgery may just postpone the inevitable. Some experts estimate that two in three tubal surgeries will move on to IVF. Unless your problem is in the proximal area and you are young (under 35), IVF may be your best bet.

See: Blocked tubes

81. ZYGOTE INTRAFALLOPIAN TRANSFER (ZIFT): Can you explain this technique? How does it differ from IVF?

Once you have agreed to a diagnostic laparoscopy, if male factor is an issue, you may consider pairing this procedure with ZIFT in order to take advantage of an opportunity to encourage conception. ZIFT, which was introduced in Australia in the late 1980s, begins with the same ovarian stimulation protocol required for IVF in the development of multiple eggs. Egg retrieval follows, as with IVF, and the harvested oocytes are mixed with sperm in the lab. At this point treatment diverges. In this scenario the female partner needs viable healthy fallopian tubes. (If your diagnosis is blocked tubes, IVF is the one and only indicated procedure.)

Rather than wait for the fertilized egg (zygote) to divide per IVF, the transfer is made within the first 24 hours of fertilization. And rather than place the embryo in the uterus, with zygote intrafallopian transfer (ZIFT) the zygote is placed directly into the fallopian tube. If the RE allows the embryo to divide before transfer by waiting until 36 hours after fertilization, the procedure is known as TET (tubal embryo transfer). This delicate procedure requires the patient to be fully anesthetized during the operation—unlike the IVF transfer procedure, which requires only a fast-acting tranquilizer. The advantage of ZIFT (or TET) is in proof of fertilization in the case of male factor and the optimal placement of the embryo.

Does ZIFT have better results than IVF? Early opinion seemed to lean toward this option for the woman over 40 who had a bleak prognosis with IVF. However, further advances with IVF (namely, ICSI and co-culture) seem to be narrowing the margin of difference. While ZIFT allows the embryo to mimic the natural course of development by beginning its development within the fallopian tube, this plus is offset by the fact that the procedure requires a full-fledged operation. Consequently, it is less frequently applied than the other forms of ART, with fewer than a thousand procedures reported in the most current SART Report (1994 results) versus 27,000 for IVF. Yet its success rate still looks stronger at 29% while IVF lags behind at 21%.

UNCONVENTIONAL
METHODS

---

82. ALTERNATIVE THERAPIES: What nontraditional options are available to enhance my chances of conceiving naturally?
Part a) ACUPUNCTURE (Chinese Medicine): Can this technique help with conception?

Although infertility has been treated with acupuncture in conjunction with traditional Chinese medicine (TCM) in China for more than eight centuries, this form of treatment has only recently gained some measure of acceptance in our country. Unlike the Western approach, which focuses on the discrete symptom, acupuncture takes into account the whole person. By analyzing the meridians (pathways) in the body, the acupuncture practitioner can pinpoint any imbalance and correct the flow of energy (Qi) with the insertion of thin needles into the appropriate meridian.

A marriage of Western and Asian medicine has evolved over the course of the twentieth century known as integral Chinese medicine (ITCM). This blend allows for the use of ART with herbal support. Since biological age is not a factor in this philosophy, people over 40 may find an alternative based on the notion that we are ageless bodies. The success of this approach hinges on full commitment by the participants, which most likely entails some modifications in lifestyle. The protocol requires practicing specific healing exercises (Qi Kung) on a regular basis to tone up the inner organs and prepare the body for conception.

When a woman exhibits signs of good health (warm extremities, no premenstrual syndrome, normal weight, and good appetite), she is considered a good candidate. Good dental hygiene is another plus. Weekly treatment sessions over the course of three consecutive cycles are required to prime the reproductive system. Diet plays a big role as well. Salads (cold food) are not recommended, especially if body heat is an issue. Eating meat, particularly lamb, is believed to strengthen the uterus. A special herbal solution known as the Rock on Tai Mountain may complete the preconception regimen to strengthen the female organs. The name refers to the steep climb and to the prayers answered at the end of the climb up the Tai Mountain, a religious shrine like Lourdes and Mecca.

What about treatments for specific problems? In the case of unexplained infertility, the TCM practitioner may suspect a liver Qi imbalance in the woman. In other words, energy (Qi) is not flowing properly in the liver meridian, and that may be creating congestion of the reproductive organs. A pulse reading at the radial (wrist) artery will confirm this diagnosis. The pulse is a multifaceted tool in this medical system, with 12 positions on each wrist and 28 qualities per position. A thorough reading of each pulse together with an examination of the tongue and general health will offer the basis for a diagnosis.

Depending upon how deep-seated the congestion is, treatment requires a commitment of at least three cycles. The profile of a woman with liver Qi congestion may be characterized by some ambivalence about parenthood. Generally she used birth control pills for an extended period, perhaps to correct an irregular period. Now she suffers from PMS and tends to work long hours, often at a thankless job. The prescription of acupuncture once per cycle together with some herbal medications could dissipate the congestion within about six months.

Women with histories of miscarriage may find relief through treatment of the kidney Qi. Poor circulation, cold extremities, and certain dietary deficiencies characterize this syndrome. The kidney Qi controls bone, bone marrow, and blood production. A well-balanced kidney Qi ensures that the circulation will nourish the embryo, protect it, and hold it in place. Again, the antidote includes a regimen of acupuncture, herbal tonics, and diet.

Male factor may respond to Chinese herbs as well. Again, the kidney energy is the focus of treatment, with results following the third month of therapy. Although Western research is scarce on this topic, a 1987 study of 250 men in China showed acupuncture to have positive results for two thirds of the subjects. Depending on how aggressively you wish to pursue this avenue, treatment may require two 30-minute sessions per week at about $80 apiece.

If you decide to use acupuncture in concert with modern ART, find a practitioner who has been licensed by the state. To qualify for the license, the acupuncturist must pass a standard curriculum. For a list of experts in your area, contact the American Academy of Acupuncture.

See: Ten Key Fertility Contacts

Part b) COUGH SYRUP: I've heard that Robitussin can adjust the cervical mucus and enhance the possibility of getting pregnant. Is there any truth to this?

Yes, there is some medical basis to this notion. The medication guaifenesin thins nasal mucus when you have a cold. At the same time it dilutes the cervical mucus. If your mucus is thick and impassable, this change in consistency may enable the sperm to travel up into the reproductive tract.

It's worth trying this approach for a few cycles if your diagnosis is scanty or thick mucus. At the very least your nasal passages will be clear.

Part c) GUIDED IMAGERY: I have heard about this book (CREATIVE VISUALIZATION) by Shakti Gawain. Has it been applied to fertility treatment? How does this technique work?

The process of guided imagery is a form of meditation using mental snapshots to help you relax. Whether using your mind in the healing process replaces traditional Western medicine is debatable. Yet everyone has spoken to or met at least one individual who beat the odds of an illness or disorder—whether infertility or some other disease—by taking an alternative approach to the situation. That person can act as a touchstone for your spiritual journey. As long as you're exploring various avenues, this is one route that has no downside.

Perhaps encountering infertility has made you reconsider the type of lifestyle you have chosen. We healthy people follow a proscribed route until we hit a roadblock. Infertility has become that roadblock for us. The mind/body connection can be a powerful tool in helping you with treatment. Even if the physical damage can't be undone (the tubes cannot reopen, the PID be reversed, etc.), the mental boost you derive from creative visualization may enhance your outcome.

The key to Shakti Gawain's approach is to repeat affirmations that describe the scenario you wish to realize. A sample would be: "I am pregnant with a beautiful, healthy baby whom I will carry to term." To support this statement, close your eyes and imagine the fetus growing in your uterus. Take this image to the ultimate one of holding the baby. Create an "album" of images that show you in the desired role of mother. Put aside 15 minutes a day for this type of conscious daydreaming.

When combined with breathing techniques, visualization has been shown to have a calming effect on blood pressure. Especially during treatment, when highs and lows may reach extremes, the ability to close your eyes and escape to this pleasant imaginary location may help. While I was waiting to be taken to the operating room for a laparoscopy, I impressed the nurse by bringing my blood pressure down to 60/80 using visualization and deep breathing.

Don't get me wrong, those negative thoughts will not go away. But you will learn how to gain control over them. You can acknowledge the inherent fears and anxieties in starting a family and let them go. Sometimes working with a therapist is helpful in setting up a system that will work for you. In his book *Spontaneous Healing,* Dr. Andrew Weil encourages patients to dispel skepticism by finding someone who has had the same problem they do and has been healed.

Part d) HERBAL CURES: *I have heard good feedback about a Chinese herb called dong quai that is indicated for "female problems." Can you tell me where it comes from?*

Dong quai, a relative of the carrot family, is derived from the root of angelica sinensis. It is to women what ginseng is to men: an elixir of youth and sexual energy. You can take it in tablet form or drink it as a liquid diluted in a cup of warm water twice a day. (It is flavorless.) Any health food store should stock this female tonic for about $10 per bottle.

In traditional Chinese medicine dong quai has been prescribed to improve circulatory disorders. Stimulating blood flow is believed to have a positive effect on the uterus and flow of female hormones. Although no Western studies exist that support this theory, in his book *Spontaneous Healing* Dr. Andrew Weil reports that his patients with menstrual or menopausal problems have taken it with good results. In my own case I believed it enhanced treatment. I have also received testimonials from other couples who added this herb to the Western protocol and were happy with the outcome.

In some cases dong quai is recommended for men in conjunction with ginseng and ho shou wo as a winning formula to enhance sperm production. Ho shou wo (which translates as "Mr. Ho has black hair"), well known in Chinese circles, is a powerful tonic that cleanses the blood and rejuvenates the body. Possible benefits include reversing the graying process in hair follicles and recovering youthful fertility levels. It can be taken as a tea called Super Shou Wu, a flowery brew. Finding this herb may take a little more research, but it should be available from any supplier of Chinese herbal medicine.

The key to success with herbs is patience. Allow two cycles or more to elapse in order for the herbs to take effect.

Part e) **HOMEOPATHIC REMEDIES:** *The TV actress Annie Potts claims that an herbalist helped her get pregnant. I'd rather go this route before I start with the expensive high tech methods. Where do I start?*

Homeopathy is based on the notion that when the energy field within the body is off-balance, a disorder will emerge. A thorough review of your health history with a homeopathic professional will determine which specially formulated remedies will reestablish your balance. All remedies are made of diluted natural substances that are unlikely to create a toxic response.

Rather than analyze what kind of problem the patient has, this approach takes into account what kind of person has the problem. If you have a case of vaginitis, for example, your diagnosis is based on information about your personality. One of three general remedies will be prescribed on the basis of your profile: Pulsatilla (for warm-natured and warm-blooded women), Sepia (for the ambitious and independent), and Natrum muriaticum (for sensitive and independent) women. While traditional medications focus on eradicating the bacteria, the homeopathic remedy builds up the immune system to create a defense against the bacteria.

Most reputable homeopaths are medical doctors who have expanded their training to include this alternative mode of treatment. Chiropractors are sometimes licensed to practice homeopathy. Classical homeopathy as practiced in the nineteenth century by the founder of this therapy, Dr. Samuel Hahneman, has always had a steady following (especially among English royalty) despite resistance by mainstream medicine. In fact, the antipathy between physicians and homeopaths dates back to the inception of the American Institute of Homeopathy in 1844. Five years later its rival, the American Medical Association, was formally established.

Probably your local Yellow Pages are a good launchpad for your search. The National Center for Homeopathy in the Washington, D.C., metropolitan area may be able to provide you with recommendations of professionals in your area or educational material that may give you some direction.

See: Ten Key Fertility Contacts

PART V

CONCERNS

WHAT IS THE CURRENT MEDICAL WISDOM ON THE SUBJECT OF . . .

83. ABORTION: *If I had an abortion 15 years ago, could there have been any damage to my reproductive organs that is preventing me from getting pregnant now?*

How vividly I recall a conversation about terminated pregnancies past in which a friend asked me, "Do you think that was our only chance to become mothers?" Certainly there are patients in fertility treatment today who may be asking themselves this very question.

Without a doubt, abortion is a subject that is bound to evoke mixed feelings if you're having trouble conceiving now. Somehow the fact that you got pregnant once gives you a false sense of confidence that you are fertile and will be able to conceive at will. But that was then, this is many years later, and in the scheme of your reproductive life, fertility is on the wane. Difficulty with conceiving is not necessarily the result of a past abortion as much as it may be a natural part of the aging process.

Yet the nagging thought may still remain: Did that abortion do permanent harm? In theory, no. A clinical abortion should not affect your reproductive system. These days the procedure, which takes place before Week 12 of gestation, is performed via suction. Provided that no complications ensue, your fertility should remain unimpaired. But as with all medical procedures, there are no guarantees. During the two weeks following the procedure, since the uterus is dilated, it is more vulnerable to infection. The introduction of bacteria can result in pelvic inflammatory disease (PID), which could diminish fertility. In order to prevent infection, the doctor will recommend no bathing, swimming, or sexual activity until after menstruation resumes.

Another complication albeit a rare one, Asherman's syndrome, may ensue if the uterine walls were scraped too vigorously during the procedure. This syndrome is characterized by scar tissue inside the uterus that may interfere with carrying a pregnancy. Repair surgery together with hormone therapy may restore the uterine lining to its original integrity. In cases of advanced age, however, IVF may have a better prognosis.

If you are concerned about postabortion complications, share your thoughts with your reproductive endocrinologist from the start of your treatment. Any adhesion inside the uterus should be obvious on the hysterosalpingogram, which would help in making your diagnosis. Don't allow self-recriminations to prevent you from getting appropriate treatment now that you are ready to have a family. Ask your RE for a referral to a psychotherapist if you need short-term counseling to help you over this hurdle.

84. AGE LIMITATION: *Recently I had a consultation with a fertility clinic that turned me away because I'm over 40. Is it my fault that I got married only last year? Is there any program that will accept my case?*

Yes, there are some women in this age group who have responded well to treatment and been able to produce take-home babies. Every practice has some small degree of success with its over 40 patients. But these happy endings are in the minority. The American Society for Reproductive Medicine is trying to get the word out: Start your families while you're young, preferably under 35. With the biological odds of becoming pregnant naturally over age 40 hovering at 5%, medical wisdom is trying to disabuse women of the notion that putting career ahead of children is feasible in the long run. Experts agree that women are not being made aware that delaying motherhood may leave no choice. Programs that treat older women do exist, but the recommended course may not be the one you had in mind.

Current research confirms that IVF success rates plummet around your 44th birthday. In other words, the quality of the eggs produced by the ovaries at that age does not make a viable embryo. For the best IVF results in the older couple, the donor egg is the way to go. In other words, you need eggs produced by a woman of prime fertility (early thirties or less). Her egg in combination with your partner's sperm will be more likely to implant. Medically your uterus may be rejuvenated with hormones that will create a receptive environment. If you want a baby—not necessarily a biological child—the odds that the donor egg will work for you are as high as six in 10 at some fertility centers.

Certainly I subscribed to the baby boom lifestyle that set the pursuit of higher education above nesting. I fully believed that I could postpone motherhood until the ripe old age of 39, which in my view was the outside limit. (A lucky hunch!) Women between 30 and 44 account for about one quarter of first-time births, according to the National Center for Health Statistics, supporting the waiting trend. Politically and financially this sequence of events makes sense. But biologically it's a gamble with consequences that cannot always be fixed by modern science. While the field of ART has made huge strides, as my doctor told me, age is not a correctable factor.

Yes, it was my good fortune to marry young enough to pursue ART successfully. And it is unfortunate that newlyweds over 40 have to find out at this juncture that biological motherhood may not be an option. Where do older eggs go wrong? Over time their integrity deteriorates, and this increases chromosomal disorders (aneuploidy). According to a study at the NYU Medical Center, a mere 9% of embryos from women 25 to 39 exhibited aneuploidies versus 42% in the group over 39. More discouraging is the fact that even "healthy" embryos may be found defective under closer scrutiny; pregenetic diagnostic testing using FISH found chromosomal problems in the "good" embryos of older patients. Could this be the key to why IVF success rates are so low? Very possibly.

What can a woman of 40 do? Consider donor egg IVF. You may have a younger relative who will volunteer her eggs, or your fertility program may have a donor. While this route may not match your image of motherhood, it is an option that is available to you even after menopause. As an insightful 43-year-old career woman told me, without a trace of bitterness, "I worked my way up the corporate ladder for 20 years to establish my career so that I could spend my hard-won earnings on having a family through donor egg IVF."

85. ALLERGIES AND DRUG REACTIONS: *I am sensitive to medication as a rule and am leery of taking chances. What are the typical side effects I may have to face if I take fertility drugs?*

Side effects of Pergonal begin with the obvious reaction to daily injections: soreness at the site of the shots.

To minimize this inevitable development, you should alternate which hip receives the shot. Of course the idea of receiving an injection is often more stressful than the actual shot. The pinch is thankfully brief. If blood appears in the syringe, you have hit a vein and must start again with a new needle. I strongly recommend applying a hot compress to the area immediately afterward. (A washcloth will do.) The heat helps disperse the drug and counteracts residual soreness the next day. Massaging the area will also help relieve discomfort as well as encourage the muscle tissue to absorb the medication.

Another common side effect is a distended belly, completely painless, as the ovaries may become somewhat enlarged. Loose waistbands are *de rigueur* during treatment. The most serious side effect, ovarian hyperstimulation syndrome, results from swollen ovaries in response to the medication. About 1% of cases require hospitalization because of fluid retention in the chest and abdomen. The balance of patients recover in the next day or two as the drug wears off. From experience I can vouch to the discomfort this entails, registering as pressure and cramps in the pelvis. But after the production of so many follicles, it is not surprising to have a degree of abdominal distress.

In general, the reaction to Pergonal may feel as familiar as premenstrual syndrome (PMS) with symptoms like moodiness, breast tenderness, and aches. You may notice excess vaginal discharge caused by accelerated mucus production by the cervix.

As for Clomid, many of the side effects from it are related to headaches and eyestrain. Headaches, dizziness, sensitivity to light, and even insomnia have been reported as possible reactions. (I experienced eye trouble to the extent that I wondered if it was time for a visit to the optometrist.) Other women report trouble in the pelvic region, stomach upset, or symptoms commonly linked to PMS, such as bloated breasts or moodiness. Ovarian cysts may appear in some women from mild overstimulation.

Internal reactions may complicate treatment. While Clomid has a good influence on ovulation, it may adversely affect the quality of cervical mucus because it keeps estrogen away from the cervix. If the mucus turns into a thick, dry paste, it may immobilize the sperm and make fertilization impossible. A postcoital test will confirm whether this is happening. Low-dose estrogen therapy for about four days following Clomid may be required to restore the proper consistency of the mucus, or your doctor may recommend intrauterine insemination.

86. BIRTH DEFECTS FOLLOWING TREATMENT: *All this laboratory intervention and the handling of embryos worry me. Are there studies about the incidence of birth defects in IVF and GIFT babies?*

Since the field of assisted reproductive technology (ART) is so young, studies examining the health of the resulting offspring are in the works. If Louise Brown, the original test-tube baby, who was born in England in 1981, represents a standard, the prognosis is excellent.

According to the most current research, birth defects among children born of artificially induced pregnancies are comparable to those conceived naturally. In other words, the difficulty in getting pregnant does not appear to translate into complications after birth. An estimated 3% of all newborns, or about 1,000 of the 34,000 ART babies born worldwide since the introduction of these technologies, exhibit birth defects.

Thankfully, the news is encouraging. At the 1996 annual meeting of the American Society for Reproductive Medicine, a symposium on this subject reported no negative impact of IVF status in a long-term study in the state of Victoria, Australia. More than 300 two-year-olds participated in this study at the Monash Medical Center. The only category where the IVF group diverged from the control was in exhibiting a greater mean length percentile: They're taller. Problems inherent to multiple or premature births were not due to medical intervention per se, since the same developments were noted among the control group. The researchers did note, however, that results may be skewed by the fact that all the participants were affluent people since socioeconomic status is a strong determining factor in the health of children.

Although these data may offer some degree of comfort to the couple leery of treatment, it's just the beginning of a long process of observation, evaluation, and analysis by the medical community. Certainly efforts will be made to resolve the issue of multiple pregnancy through ART in order to reduce the number of premature babies. But for the patient who needs to make a decision right now, medical science offers you tentative optimism.

87. CANCELED CYCLES (*Hypothalamic Pituitary Disorder*): *After I took a course of fertility drugs, my doctor said I wasn't responding well. Apparently I produced only two small eggs. Consequently he called off the procedure, which I found quite upsetting. Does this mean that my case is hopeless? I am 36.*

How you respond to fertility drugs is the key to your treatment and prognosis. If your body produces only a couple of immature ova during a medicated cycle, the inference is that you have a hypothalamic pituitary disorder that is interfering with timely ovulation. In other words, signals between the hypothalamus (the midportion of the brain) and the pituitary gland are not cooperating to release female hormones according to the monthly timetable. Without the proper flow of female hormones Pergonal will not be able to do its magic.

If a cycle is called off or canceled for lack of response, your RE will reassess your situation. Further analysis will reveal whether you may have polycystic ovarian syndrome, the condition most closely associated with hypothalamic pituitary disorder, or a thyroid condition. Either diagnosis can be controlled and treated with further medications.

When additional tests uncover elevated follicle-stimulating hormone (FSH), the indication is that your ovaries are entering the shutdown mode. No fertility drug can reverse signs of ovarian failure, which is not to be confused with hypothalamic pituitary failure. In the latter condition, menstruation has followed a sporadic, unpredictable course following puberty. Sometimes small tumors sitting on the pituitary are responsible for the short circuit in hormone production. As they grow, these tumors may cause headaches or eye problems. Again, proper medication can shrink these otherwise harmless growths and restore fertility. Unless you are in ovarian failure, a single canceled cycle may not mean the end of treatment.

88. CHEMICAL PREGNANCY (Positive *h*CG): In the clinic I have heard the nurses speak of chemical pregnancies. From what I understand it's a false reading of some sort, which sounds discouraging. Can you explain?

If you don't get your period on the expected date following a cycle of fertility treatment, you may be pregnant. For IVF patients a beta hCG blood pregnancy test may be scheduled only nine days following the embryo transfer, well before the next cycle would begin. If the test comes back positive, you have a chemical pregnancy, which means you have an elevated level of hCG. That is good news by implication since it could mean that the embryo is implanting. (A less desirable explanation for elevated hCG may be the presence of tumors.) Two days later you will repeat the blood test. If the embryo implantation is going well, the hCG level should have doubled.

Once the presence of the fetus has been confirmed through ultrasound, you have graduated to a clinical pregnancy. Keep in mind that an estimated one quarter of all naturally conceived pregnancies don't progress from the chemical stage. Complicating matters for the woman in IVF treatment is the fact that hCG is part of the protocol. Although the hCG injection is administered about 10 days prior to the pregnancy test, unabsorbed levels of the drug in the bloodstream could yield a false-positive reading. In no case should chemical pregnancy be construed to mean a full-fledged clinical pregnancy as a measure of success rates.

89. CLINIC MISTAKES: *One of my friends who was in in vitro treatment had an embarrassing event happen that canceled her cycle. A nurse accidentally walked in on her husband while he was trying to produce a specimen, and he lost his erection. Is the clinic liable in such a situation? . . . Could a doctor accidentally transfer the wrong embryos into a patient? . . . With insemination can I be guaranteed that my husband's sperm is being used?*

Human error is always a factor when dealing with people, and the field of ART is no exception. But it is an extremely rare occurrence. No matter how small the margin of error, these mistakes have enormous repercussions for both patients and clinics. When a white couple in Scandinavia had twins, one of whom was black, the situation was traced back to a pipette that hadn't been properly cleaned before reuse. In California another scandal erupted when the embryos of more than two dozen patients at the Center for Reproductive Health at Irvine were given away without their consent. And what about the doctors who donate their own sperm to patients in need?

In order to protect consumers, new regulations have been formulated by the American Medical Association's Division of Ethics and Standards. The Society for Assisted Reproductive Technology (SART) has also initiated new policies, including a release consent form that must be signed by patients who retain complete control over their genetic material.

In 1995 the American Society for Reproductive Medicine (ASRM) issued a statement regarding its commitment to the safe and effective care of fertility patients and to enforcing the ethical practice guidelines as set by its affiliates. While the ASRM acknowledges that unethical behavior cannot be entirely eradicated, membership in its organization requires adherence to its high standard of treatment.

If proved mishandling occurs in your case, you have grounds to demand a refund or its equivalent. Certainly, if a cycle is canceled because of sample interruptus, the clinic should take responsibility. As for swapping embryos or sperm samples, it behooves the clinic to have good lab controls in place in order to contain legal fees. In a field where word of mouth recommendations are worth their weight in gold, no professional wishes to jeopardize the reputation of the program. If you don't trust your RE or the staff to use the sperm sample you supplied, then perhaps it's time to find a new practice. As long as your specialist is a member of the ASRM, you may feel that every measure is being taken to ensure that you will receive the best care.

90. ECTOPIC (TUBAL) PREGNANCY: *I've heard that IVF increases the odds of tubal pregnancy. Is this true?*

For the average woman of reproductive age, the odds of having an ectopic pregnancy are about 1%. The number doubles for the woman with a fertility problem and doubles again to 4% following embryo transfer. Despite the fact that IVF occurs in a hospital environment, the risk of an embryo's going off course cannot be eliminated entirely. About 3% of IVF patients will face termination of a clinical pregnancy that has implanted improperly somewhere in the reproductive system other than the uterus. Unless you take swift action, internal bleeding or rupturing of the tube may put your life in jeopardy.

The fallopian tubes are a pair of delicate, narrow vessels about four inches long that connect the ovaries to the uterus. Protrusions that act as fingers (fimbriae) carry the egg from the ovary and guide it into the uterus. The diameter of the tube is minuscule, and that is why it is so easily obstructed. Once you learn of a blockage, the natural reaction is to have the obstruction removed so that the function may return to normal. Who wouldn't prefer to conceive under natural circumstances? The best candidates for tubal repair surgery are women with healthy tubes that are blocked at the proximal or fimbriated end. Unfortunately this group represents only a small segment of those with tubal blockage.

What you should know is that the chance of an ectopic (tubal) pregnancy may actually increase following tubal surgery. The reason is that residual scarring leads the embryo to implant outside the uterus. As the catheter releases the embryos, the liquid may wash them into the fallopian tubes rather than into the uterus.

Fortunately, IVF patients are being monitored so closely that corrective action can be taken before the tube ruptures. If the hCG levels are high, yet no fetus is visible on the ultrasound monitor, the situation begins to reveal itself. The patient may experience some pelvic cramping or vaginal bleeding. Unfortunately, today's technology does not have the capability of transferring the embryo back into the uterus. Instead the embryo must be removed surgically or absorbed into the body through a fast-acting prescription drug (methotrexate).

91. FROZEN EMBRYOS—DELAYED TRANSFERS:
What are the success rates on thawing frozen embryos? It all sounds so brave new world to me. . . . What happens to "extra" frozen embryos if you have a successful pregnancy with the first transfer? Is it costly to store them? How long do they "keep"?

The 1996 SART Report cites 15% success with the transfer of frozen embryos, 10 years after this technique was introduced in Australia. With superovulation typically creating a surfeit of embryos and a ceiling of four embryos per transfer, the prospect of banking any extra is a boon. For couples who produce more than six to eight viable embryos, the appeal is two for the price of one; freezing may prove to be cost-effective since a single retrieval may produce two pregnancies. And as thawing techniques improve, with 80% of embryos surviving, fertility practitioners are reconsidering the role of cryopreservation in the big picture. Revised opinion views freezing no longer as just a storage technique for excess embryos but as a viable method with good success rates that may be the wave of the future.

What new developments have changed attitudes? First, a gentler chemical (propanediol) is now in use to preserve the integrity of the embryos. In the early 1990s up to one third of cryopreserved embryos did not survive thawing after storage. Secondly, it has been discovered that freezing the embryos as soon as possible may yield better results. Development in the lab petri dish seems to have better results when it takes place after thawing, instead of beforehand, as was the case.

For the patient who responds well to fertility drugs, the benefits of cryopreservation are clear: You may produce enough embryos in one cycle for two or more transfers. Depending upon the program, the frozen transfer occurs during a natural cycle at the time of your choice. Some practitioners prefer to prepare the uterus with female hormones. Does all this mechanical handling harm the embryo? On the contrary, in an illustration of Darwinian theory, survival of the fittest seems to rule on the issues of freezing and thawing.

The lab will bill you for storage of the embryos while they remain in a frozen state. How long will they "keep"? The technique is too new to gauge, although there are recorded cases of a pregnancy following five years of cryopreservation. Depending upon the results of the initial transfer, most women return for frozen transfers within months of retrieval. For women who conceive with the first transfer, pregnancy will delay the return. I do know of women who have gone on to successful second pregnancies from the same harvest, essentially giving birth to fraternal "twins" with completely different birthdays and birth years.

92. GOVERNMENT REGULATION (LEGAL PARAMETERS): How are fertility programs being regulated, if at all?

This field is self-regulated through the efforts of the American Society of Reproductive Medicine (ASRM). Practitioners are kept up-to-date on the latest technology and techniques at an annual convention. In addition, its publication, *Fertility and Sterility,* ongoing conferences, and seminars held year-round help keep specialists apprised of new developments, which continue to be introduced at a rapid pace.

Although the Fertility Clinic Success Rate and Certification Act was passed by Congress in 1992, at the urging of Representative Ron Wyden (D-Oregon), little has ensued because of the lack of federal funds. As the situation stands now, the collection of data from participating clinics is being handled by the Society for Assisted Reproductive Technology (SART), a branch of the ASRM, which publishes the SART Report on a biannual basis. In the future, a committee drawing representatives from four groups—the ASRM, the Centers for Disease Control and Prevention, and Resolve, the infertility patient advocacy group, and SART—will collaborate to establish guidelines for the definition of pregnancy success rates. Clinics will be required to list which embryo labs they use and whether the labs are certified by the Reproductive Lab Accreditation Program of the College of American Pathologists. An annual report will be issued under CDC auspices to update success rates, identify which lab is associated with each participating clinic, and list nonparticipating clinics. Finally, the CDC will set a standard for lab certification based on the Reproductive Lab Accreditation Program. While the law allows the government to conduct unscheduled lab visits, the CDC hasn't followed through. Setting up the checks and balances is a tedious and expensive proposition.

Government research on the subject of in vitro and implantation is under way meanwhile at the National Institutes of Health. In 1996 a group of experts formed the Human Embryo Research Panel (aka the National Bioethics Advisory Commission) to address the scientific and ethical issues inherent to this new medical field. The FDA is attempting to set some standards, with special attention to the handling of donor gametes. On the legal front the American Bar Association's Laws of Reproduction and Genetic Technology Committee is drafting model legislation to help set some guidelines in four areas: access, gametes and embryos, clinical standards, and oversight and enforcement.

93. HIGH-RISK PREGNANCY: *Once I am pregnant, will I require special care because I conceived through ART?*

Not necessarily. Having trouble getting pregnant does not imply that your pregnancy is at risk unless you have a structural problem like a tipped uterus. In fact, I was the first IVF pregnancy that my obstetrician had ever handled, and he had received his degree in 1949. Once my fertility doctor released my case, I wanted to blend into the fertile world. Then again, I found my obstetrician by calling a member of Resolve who had recently given birth.

94. HYPERSTIMULATED OVARIES: *My doctor explained that Pergonal therapy can affect the ovaries adversely. In the clinic I've spoken to other women who have experienced discomfort following retrieval. Are there long-term effects I should know about? What causes this syndrome?*

In a word, Pergonal (hMG). As many as one in five women may experience mild symptoms of abdominal discomfort or bloating while on the medication. Since your ovaries may produce an astonishing number of follicles, anywhere from three up to 30 or more, a physical reaction is not too surprising. But for a small group—about 1%—the reaction can become serious. This is why constant monitoring is so crucial to Pergonal therapy.

As the fertility drug cultivates the follicles to maturity, your ovaries may swell or "weep" with the effort, and you may notice bloating in your abdomen. Other signals of potential hyperstimulation are elevated estrogen levels or pelvic discomfort, such as cramps. In extremely rare cases the accumulation of fluid in the abdomen or chest may cause sudden distension or interfere with breathing.

Because Pergonal is such a powerful drug, each patient is closely followed with blood tests and ultrasound. By checking your levels daily during the course of treatment, your reproductive endocrinologist can assess how your body is reacting to the fertility drug and make decisions based on latest readings. If you are considered at risk for hyperstimulation, your doctor may elect to cancel the cycle by forgoing the hCG injection, and that puts a halt to ovulation. While aborting treatment may be discouraging, what has been gained is the information about your body. In a future cycle Pergonal dosage can then be adjusted for better results.

In selected cases doctors may be able to salvage the hyperstimulated cycle with a new technique called prolonged coasting. This method, introduced by the Pacific Fertility Medical Centers, adds another fertility drug to the mix: GnRHa, commercially sold as Lupron or Synarel. When the female hormone estradiol soars, Lupron replaces Pergonal until the level settles down. Once the doctor thinks that hormone levels are within a safe range, the green light is given for the hCG injection.

95. PHOBIAS—FEAR OF MEDICAL TREATMENT:
Before I found out I was infertile, going to the doctor was the last thing I'd ever do. Now that I'm faced with possible surgery and the prospect of injections, self-administered no less, I am feeling seriously stressed out. How can I overcome these fears so that I can go on with treatment?

If deep breathing or relaxation techniques don't work for you, perhaps some short-term counseling will. Behavioral modification therapy, such as consciously replacing an anxious thought with a beautiful image, may help in the immediate situation. In extreme cases of anxiety, hypnosis may help you over the hurdle of entering the operating room. Most fertility programs either have psychotherapists on staff or can make referrals. Each step of the way fertility treatment is a test of your mettle and your commitment to the process. Respect your limits. If an invasive procedure like a laparoscopy oversteps your personal boundaries, you may stop treatment there and explore other avenues.

Since the fertility pill (Clomid) is indicated for the ovulation factor, if your diagnosis falls outside that proscribed factor, you will soon be faced with human menopausal gonadotropin (hMG) therapy. As a protein hMG would be broken down by the digestive system if taken orally, and that would render it powerless. Instead it must be given intramuscularly with a sturdy needle in the privacy of your home.

You will learn the difference between subcutaneous injections and intramuscular ones. Often Metrodin therapy is preceded by Lupron, which means also using a needle, albeit a small, thin one that can be self-administered even by the otherwise queasy. Who would ever imagine herself buying a bag of syringes at the local pharmacy? A woman faced with tubal factor infertility, for one. Your clinic will fully and clearly demonstrate technique beforehand. Pergonal and Metrodin, in powder form, need to be prepared with a liquid (often saline). You dip the needle into the liquid, then into the powder. Once the syringe is ready, the needle is usually given in the upper quadrant of the hip. Again, you may now request Fertinex instead, available in the U.S. as of 1996.

Not every partner can step to the plate on administering this treatment, and there are alternatives. For example, you can hire a nurse to help you through the course of treatment (a few weeks at most). Look beyond your mate for help if he can't handle this aspect of treatment. Is there a friend or neighbor you can trust with this responsibility? Even if you manage to replace the Metrodin prescription with Fertinex, it is usually followed by progesterone, which could mean injections for anywhere from two weeks to two months (if you get lucky).

96. PREGNANCY LOSS—MISCARRIAGE AND ECTOPIC PREGNANCY: *After losing one pregnancy, I worry about losing the next one. Yet I've heard of women who lost several pregnancies and went on to have healthy babies. How can I dispel these worries? Are there statistics that show the success rates following pregnancy loss?*

Four out of 10 women with histories of two or even three miscarriages will go on to carry a baby to term without any medical intervention whatsoever. While one miscarriage may enhance the odds of another, a past full-term pregnancy may increase the odds for another success especially if you're under 35. For those over 35, the incidence of miscarriage becomes more common because of chromosomal abnormalities associated with older gametes. In fact, an estimated half of all early miscarriages are due to a genetic defect.

From experience I can testify to the crash from elation to despair that ensues when a pregnancy does not go to term. In my case the psychological healing process took six months before I was ready to return to treatment and risk another disappointment. Even though the odds of a repeat ectopic pregnancy were slim since one tube had been removed and the other closed off, the remote chance haunted me. Grieving is part of the process of recovery, particularly following the rigors of fertility treatment. For me, short-term enrollment in a support group helped me through this rough patch.

The temptation to worry about a recurrence is to be expected, and every action may become suspect. Although there is no guarantee that it won't happen again, the underlying pathology is more likely to be related to uterine or hormonal abnormalities, or structural problems within the embryo, rather than to your physical actions. About one in six women will be diagnosed with a structural problem of the uterus. Next in line your RE will check for thyroid problems or luteal phase deficiency, which can be corrected through medication.

Experts agree that in the early weeks of pregnancy you may follow your normal routine (provided that you're not an Olympic athlete) without risking loss. Elevating your legs is not a preventive measure. And to date neither exposure to computers nor hair dye has been proved to interfere with proper fetal development. Nor are venereal infections responsible for miscarriage; rather, they are linked to tubal factor infertility.

What may put your next pregnancy in jeopardy during your first trimester is smoking or drinking or nonfertility prescription drugs. Most fertility patients are conscientious about inquiring about the possible impact of other medications on current treatment. For about 5% of couples with recurrent miscarriage a diagnosis of genetic abnormality may indicate a higher risk of loss. The abnormality is identified by analysis of fetal tissue (where available) or by blood tests for both partners. Since not all abnormalities result in recurrent loss, you may need to sit down with a genetic counselor to review your risks and weigh the options.

Your doctor may recommend a course of progesterone as a preventive measure throughout the first trimester. Natural progesterone (in injection or suppository form), which is secreted by the ovary following ovulation, builds up the uterine lining to encourage implantation. What are the repercussions of this drug on the developing embryo? Nothing adverse has been observed. Since it is administered in small doses in its natural form, progesterone may be safely taken through week nine of gestation.

97. SELECTIVE REDUCTION—MULTIPLES: At the beginning of treatment I used to fantasize about having twins. But now that I have some friends who have twins I'm less eager for this outcome. In fact, at my program I have heard about women who conceived triplets and were relieved to have lost an embryo or two. I understand that the doctor can reduce the number of embryos surgically. Financially we couldn't handle two children at this time. How does selective reduction work?

When you are exerting every effort to conceive and carry a baby to term, a multiple pregnancy is an exciting possibility. You may think of twins as a boon, a shortcut to building that dream family with two children. Multiples help erase the stigma of infertility forever; you may feel renewed and vindicated.

But the reality of carrying two or more healthy babies for 40 weeks may temper your initial rush of enthusiasm. Especially in the case of triplets or more, the potential for complications or miscarriage increases sharply. Sometimes to ensure that a single healthy one will be born, your doctor will recommend that you reduce the number of embryos at the outset. Before 12 weeks of gestation a chemical injection would eliminate excess embryos, which would be absorbed into the body. The dominant embryo would continue to develop to term.

You may wonder, isn't that abortion? Technically, perhaps. But under the circumstances it is viewed as protection against a high-risk or lost pregnancy. Multiple pregnancies present a danger to the mother with serious implications, such as high blood pressure or uterine bleeding. While experts are striving to refine ART in order to eliminate or at least to contain the possibility of multiples, right now it cannot be ruled out. Multifetal selective reduction may not be the ideal solution to successful treatment, but it offers an alternative.

If this scenario concerns you, discuss the odds with your doctor. Set limits on how many embryos will be transferred per cycle. Find out how many sets of triplets or quads have been produced at the practice. But don't allow this concern to stop your treatment from making progress.

PART VI

RESOURCES

WHERE TO FIND MEDICAL REFERRALS

98. FERTILITY TREATMENT PROGRAMS: Where are the best clinics?

The official source for referrals is the 50-plus-year-old American Society for Reproductive Medicine (formerly the American Fertility Society), a nonprofit organization based in Birmingham, Alabama, and the publisher of the famous SART Report. Its 10,000 members collaborate to produce *Fertility and Sterility*, a monthly scientific journal reporting the latest studies from the field. They also produce educational brochures for free distribution to the universe of fertility patients on issues pertinent to treatment.

Within the ASRM there are three subdivisions: the Society of Reproductive Endocrinologists (SRE), the Society of Reproductive Surgeons (SRS), and the Society for Assisted Reproductive Technology (SART). Every two years this latter affiliate updates the SART Report, complete with statistical data from 250 member fertility clinics citing success rates by region. Since the process of compiling data is time-consuming, statistics in the current issue may be slightly out-of-date. Still, it will give you some direction on the clinic that might be best equipped to treat your case. Since the SART Report is costly ($45), you may be able to consult it at or borrow it from a local medical library. With thousands of specialists throughout the country, narrowing your choice to one seems daunting at first. But once you have a diagnosis, it will facilitate the selection process.

How reliable are the statistics? Although the ASRM strives to create standard measures, there is some controversy about how success rates are calculated. Some clinics may appear more successful than others, but on closer inspection you will see that they are treating a younger population to ensure the higher degree of success. As a result, many women over 40 are being shut out of some programs just on the basis of age.

What you want to find out is the take-home-baby rate for your age bracket for couples with your diagnosis. With the current trend of rising treatment costs and diminishing health insurance coverage, the ASRM is doing its best to exert some influence on legislation. Through these efforts, the National Institutes of Health now includes two infertility research centers.

99. SPERM BANKS: How do we find a reputable one? We want to freeze sperm for future use since my husband is in chemotherapy. . . . I'm a single woman interested in having a baby. Where can I get donor sperm?

Your urologist should be able to help you find a sperm bank with good credentials in your area for safekeeping until future use. Or the ASRM can provide you with a list. With more than 400 sperm banks in business in our country, availability is surprising. Who monitors these facilities? Depending on state laws, some localities issue licenses while others impose no controls at all.

When interviewing a sperm bank, inquire if the guidelines of the American Association of Tissue Banks are being enforced. Since compliance is not required by law, it is recommended and would indicate that the facility is responsible. If you are looking for a donor, investigate the bank's screening policies: Does it take a thorough medical history for each donor? Has it recorded all hereditary medical conditions? Does it freeze and quarantine semen for at least six months and follow up to test for HIV? Clearly, the answer to this last question is crucial. Prior to 1985 donors were not tested for HIV, and this failure led to infection in a small percentage of recipients. Since then the six-month quarantine has become mandatory, and no further cases have been reported.

Another consideration is disclosure. In the past, sperm donors were completely anonymous and expected to stay that way. But the climate changed in 1989, when Sweden introduced a new policy of open identity; information about the biological father will become available upon request once the child reaches its majority as of the year 2007. Nowadays this trend toward openness has spread to the United States, beginning with the Sperm Bank of California in Berkeley. Depending upon the recipient's comfort level, privacy may be another criterion when selecting a donor.

100. VOLUNTEER SERVICES (HOT LINE SUPPORT): Can I call someone about doctor referrals?

If you're experiencing information overload on this subject, as does happen, maybe it's time to reach out to someone who's been there, done that. Sharing your thoughts with someone who has experienced treatment may be just what the doctor ordered. From my experience, I would recommend Resolve. For more than two decades this nonprofit organization run by member volunteers has provided education and support to the infertile population. Why the name? To reflect its mission as a clearinghouse to help members come to grips with and *resolve* feelings and issues that accompany this life crisis. Although the national headquarters are located in Boston, Resolve has chapters in all 50 states. In addition to a quarterly newsletter, annual membership entitles you to attend monthly meetings, participate in support groups, and make telephone contact.

For me Resolve offered direction and clarification during the difficult times of treatment. Like most members, I learned about the group through literature at the doctor's office. Once I "resolved" my situation through a successful IVF cycle, I signed up with the hot line. All messages are recorded by an answering machine for callback by a trained volunteer within three days. While the majority of callers are seeking doctor referrals or insurance advice, others want to connect specifically with people who share their diagnoses. Resolve can help on all counts.

If you're looking for conferences or workshops pertaining to your treatment, contact the Ferre Institute, which is another nonprofit group dedicated to fertility research and education. Ferre often collaborates with Resolve to sponsor meetings of interest to fertility patients.

See: Ten Key Fertility Contacts

101. INTERNET: *Where can I find on-line information?*

All hot line resources may be accessed through the World Wide Web. You will find hundreds of sites under the heading of "infertility," including chat rooms on various aspects of treatment. Many fertility programs advertise their services through the Internet.

Here are five handpicked Web sites that may offer

you specific answers and help with the issues yo.
facing right now:

1. Fertility Information Resource List
   http://www.vais.net/-travis/firl.html

2. INCIID (InterNational Council for Infertility
   Information Dissemination)
   http://www.inciid.org

This educational group, established in 1994 by
three women in treatment, is dedicated to offering
the consumer the latest on-line technological fertility
bulletins at no cost. INCIID has launched an on-line
survey of people who visit its site in order to measure
the scope of infertility and serve as a model for
health care providers. Results are expected to be
available when you read this. All three cofounders
gave birth in 1995, two on the same day.

3. Donor Egg IVF Support Groups
   http://www.ihr.com/resolve/donor.html

4. Donor Sperm
   http://www.mindspnng.com/-xytex/issues.html

5. Resolve
   http://www.resolve.org

AFTERWORD

MY STORY: Did treatment work for me?

Yes, ultimately and frustratingly, after five years of working with various doctors and following some blind alleys before coming up with the definitive diagnosis of blocked tubes. Once the problem was identified as tubal damage, it turned out I was an ideal candidate for IVF. The quality of sperm and eggs was good, and my uterus was in working order. Above all, what I had on my side was time: I entered treatment on the eve of my 35th birthday, on the threshold of the slippery downward spiral. Working with the five-year window, I allowed myself the luxury of scheduling treatments with big breaks in between.

My only regret is that I spent too much time spinning my wheels with an ordinary gynecologist while in my early thirties. At the time I consulted this man, the concept of fertility treatment was fairly new. Month after month I brought in temperature charts like homework for his review. He would critique the timing of our sexual activity (not enough, too much, on the wrong day). When I mentioned that the time might have come for more aggressive action, this physician had the audacity to accuse me of being impatient and looking for instant results, a character flaw of my generation as a whole! If you feel frustrated with your current doctor, put this book down and find another doctor *this instant.*

GLOSSARY

ACID TYRODE'S DIGESTION Form of assisted hatching whereby the zona (egg cover) is partially eroded by a chemical solution.

ACROSOME Sperm's head cover, which plays a crucial role in penetration of the egg by releasing enzymes that promote fertilization.

ADENOMYOSIS Uterine condition characterized by the abnormal growth of endometrial glands on the uterine wall and possible painful periods.

ALLOIMMUNITY Development of antibodies in a woman's body triggered by the introduction of male proteins (sperm).

ANOVULATION Failure of the ovaries to produce an ovum.

ANTIBODIES Blood proteins set off by an immunological reaction that may deactivate an invader (in this case, sperm) by attacking them or causing them to clump in a way that renders them ineffective; and detectable through a blood test.

ANTILYMPHOCYTE ANTIBODIES (ALAs) Blood proteins in the female partner that combat lymphocytes introduced by the male partner or a growing fetus.

ANTIPHOSPHOLIPID ANTIBODIES (APAs) Blood proteins that undermine the root system of the placenta in the early stages of conception.

ART (assisted reproductive technology) Any of the various

clinical procedures that attempt to produce human embryos outside the body through combining the use of fertility drugs and surgical intervention in the pursuit of pregnancy.

ARTIFICIAL INSEMINATION   The insertion of chemically treated sperm into the vagina or uterus via catheter in a fertility practitioner's office.

ASHERMAN'S SYNDROME   Scar tissue in the uterine cavity associated with surgery.

ASRM   The American Society for Reproductive Medicine, the professional group that represents this specialization.

ASSISTED HATCHING   A chemical treatment applied to a human egg prior to fertilization in the IVF process in which the zona pellucida (outer shell) is thinned prior to embryo transfer.

ASSISTED REPRODUCTIVE TECHNOLOGY   See ART.

AUTOIMMUNE DISORDER   Possible cause of miscarriage when a woman's body creates antibodies that reject the embryo as a foreign body.

BASAL BODY TEMPERATURE (BBT)   A measure of ovulation as reflected by a woman's temperature over the course of 28 days.

BILLINGS METHOD   A measure of ovulation using cervical mucus secretions.

BIOPSY   A diagnostic test that requires the analysis of a small piece of an organ, such as the endometrium (uterine lining).

CAPACITATION   Transformation in a sperm cell as it travels through the female reproductive system that precedes fertilization of an egg.

CERVICAL MUCUS   A vaginal secretion resembling egg whites that signals ovulation in mid-cycle—and a troublemaker for an estimated 10% of infertile couples.

CERVIX   The lower part of the female reproductive tract that connects the uterus with the vagina.

CHEMICAL PREGNANCY   An unconfirmed positive pregnancy blood test that shows falsely elevated levels of hCG.

CLINICAL PREGNANCY   A positive pregnancy test confirmed by ultrasound.

CLOMID (clomiphene citrate)   The fertility "pill" prescribed to regulate ovulation.

CLOMIPHENE CITRATE   See preceding entry.

CO-CULTURE   An IVF technique whereby tissue from either human or bovine fallopian tubes is added to the medium in the petri dish.

CONTROLLED SUPEROVULATION (enhanced follicular recruitment/controlled ovarian hyperstimulation)   The process of stimulating the ovaries through the use of ovulation drugs (such as Pergonal, Metrodin, and Humegon) in order to produce a large crop of eggs during a menstrual cycle.

CRYOPRESERVATION   The technique used both in storing excess embryos following IVF treatment and in storing sperm for future use. When the embryos are preserved in liquid nitrogen at 196 degrees below zero, they remain viable for several years following fertilization and may be thawed for transfer in a future attempt at pregnancy. There is no equivalent way to store eggs.

CYCLE   A measure of the ovulation process that begins with menstruation on Day 1, passes through ovulation on Day 14, and lasts between 28 and 32 days until the next period begins.

DES (diethylstilbestrol)   A prenatal drug taken by pregnant women in the 1950s and 1960s that created infertility in resulting children.

DONG QUAI   A Chinese herb associated with enhancing fertility.

DONOR EGG   The genetic material contributed by a fertile woman to a couple that requires better-quality eggs in the pursuit of IVF treatment.

DONOR EMBRYO   A viable embryo given to an infertile woman or couple in pursuit of IVF treatment.

DONOR SPERM   The genetic material in frozen form contributed by a fertile man to a sperm bank for use with ART or insemination.

ECTOPIC PREGNANCY (tubal) A pregnancy outside the uterus that must be terminated since the embryo attaches improperly, usually in the fallopian tube.

EGG (ovum/oocyte) Female genetic material the size of a grain of sand produced by the ovaries and released monthly. When combined with sperm, it forms an embryo.

EGG RETRIEVAL A half hour operating room procedure in IVF treatment following drug therapy and timed to ovulation whereby the eggs are harvested via a needle while the patient is lightly anesthetized.

EJACULATE The male semen.

EMBRYO The first stage of human life resulting from the union of egg and sperm within the first eight weeks following fertilization. Becomes a blastocyst (advanced-stage embryo).

EMBRYO TRANSFER Part of the IVF procedure when the embryo or embryos are taken from the lab petri dish and replaced vaginally into the uterus via a catheter.

ENDOCRINOLOGY The study of hormones.

ENDOMETRIAL BIOPSY Measure of ovulation using a specimen of the endometrium to pinpoint function.

ENDOMETRIOSIS A disease characterized by painful periods caused by the endometrium growing outside the uterus, which occurs most often in women who postpone childbearing.

ENDOMETRIUM The uterine lining that is expelled in the menstrual flow every month unless a pregnancy occurs.

EPIDIDYMIS Final sperm stop in the male genitals prior to ejaculation.

ESTRADIOL Female hormone produced by ovarian follicles (aka E_2).

ESTROGEN Female hormone.

FALLOPIAN TUBES A pair of small tubes that connects the ovaries to the uterus; the site of fertilization.

FERTILITY DRUGS Hormones in tablet or injection form that stimulate the ovaries to produce more than a single egg per cycle.

FERTINEX   A highly purified form of FSH, an ovulation drug.

FETUS   A developed embryo of eight weeks or more.

FIBROID TUMOR   A benign growth (fibroma) in the uterus that may interfere with fertility.

FIMBRIAE   The endmost part of the fallopian tube resembling a fringe that vacuums the ova from the ovaries.

FISH (fluorescence in-situ hybridization)   A procedure that identifies chromosomal defects, using the polar body (aka chromosome painting).

FOLLICLE   The outer shell that contains the female egg and other female sex hormones stored in the ovaries.

FSH (follicle-stimulating hormone)   A protein hormone generated by the pituitary that stimulates the ovaries to produce follicles (eggs) in women and the testicles to produce sperm in men. An FSH defect may impair fertility or cause miscarriage. Synthetically known as Metrodin and Fertinex.

GAMETE   Egg or sperm.

GIFT (gamete intrafallopian transfer)   An ART procedure that attempts pregnancy through the surgical injection of treated sperm and retrieved ova into the fallopian tubes without fertilization when the patient is under general anesthesia.

GnRHa (gonadotropin-releasing hormone antagonist)   A medication administered through injection that suspends a woman's production of female hormones. Synthetically produced as Lupron and Synarel.

GONADOTROPIN   A hormone (either LH or FSH) released by the pituitary that stimulates the ovaries or testicles.

GRAAFIAN FOLLICLE   A dominant egg during natural ovulation.

HAMSTER PENETRATION TEST   Measure of sperm's penetration ability to enter an egg, in this case of a hamster.

HATCHING   The preimplantation stage of a developing embryo.

HEPARIN   An anticlotting drug that may counter an immunological dysfunction.

HORMONE   A chemical released by the ovary or testicle that determines reproductive function.

HUMAN CHORIONIC GONADOTROPIN (hCG)   A female hormone derived from the urine of pregnant women that triggers ovulation in hMG therapy and is used as the measure in pregnancy testing.

HUMAN MENOPAUSAL GONADOTROPIN (hMG)   A powerful fertility drug derived from the urine of menopausal women that induces superovulation through carefully monitored injections. Commercially sold as Pergonal and Humegon.

HYDROSALPINX   Water on the fallopian tube caused by blockage at the fimbriated end by the ovary.

HYPERSTIMULATION   A possible side effect of hMG that causes swelling of the ovaries and a degree of physical discomfort.

HYPOSPADIA   Birth defect of the penis.

HYPOSPERMATOGENESIS   Low sperm count.

HYPOTHALAMUS   Part of the brain that regulates the release of the sex hormones (estrogen and progesterone for women and testosterone for men) that control the pituitary gland.

HYSTEROSALPINGOGRAM (HSG)   X ray of the uterus and fallopian tubes using an injection of a dye into the cervix.

HYSTEROSCOPY   Surgical exam of cervix and uterus through a hysteroscope that enables corrective action without major surgery.

ICSI (intracytoplasmic sperm injection)   Micromanipulation technique whereby a single treated sperm is injected into a mature egg to encourage fertilization.

IMPLANTATION   The stage that follows fertilization when the embryo settles into the endometrium.

IUI (intrauterine insemination)   A method of injecting chemically washed sperm into the uterus and bypassing the cervix, where hostile mucus may prevent fertilization.

IVF (in vitro fertilization)   The process of mixing a woman's eggs with a partner's sperm in a glass dish (in vitro) after fertility drug treatment and allowing embryos to develop outside the body before transferring a maximum of three or four back into the woman's uterus. Fertilization without drugs is called natural IVF.

IVI (intravaginal insemination)   Injection of sperm, most often donor sperm, into the vagina.

IVIG (intravenous immunoglobulin)   Experimental technique that suppresses "killer cells" in the woman's body with IV injections of protein substances to prevent miscarriage.

KARYOTYPE   Chromosomal profile.

LAPAROSCOPY   A diagnostic test that takes place in the operating room to measure with a scope the capability of a woman's reproductive system. An augmented laparoscopy includes an egg retrieval.

LAPAROTOMY   Major abdominal surgery, which may be required to remove abnormal growths that may obstruct fertilization.

LUTEAL PHASE (LH phase)   The half of a woman's menstrual cycle following ovulation (aka secretory phase). LH is the hormone produced by the pituitary to trigger ovulation.

LUTEAL PHASE DEFECT (LPD)   Chemical imbalance in the second half of a woman's cycle that may result in miscarriage.

METRODIN   A gonadotropin similar to Pergonal.

MICROMANIPULATION   Laboratory techniques that encourage the sperm to fertilize an egg with IVF (ICSI, PESA, ROSNI, SUZI).

MOTILITY   Measure of a sperm's ability to travel through the woman's reproductive tract.

MÜLLERIAN ANOMALY   Birth defect of the uterus.

MYCELES   Netlike fibers within the cervical mucus measured in the PCT to determine whether they are hostile or welcoming.

MYCOPLASMA   Bacteria in the cervical mucus potentially hostile to sperm.

OVARIES   The source of ovulation (ova) located on each side of the pelvis, joined to the uterus by the fallopian tubes.

OVULATION   The release of a mature egg by the ovaries at the midpoint of a woman's cycle.

OVULATION KIT   An over-the-counter test that measures the LH in a woman's urine to determine when she will ovulate.

OVUM   Female gamete about the size of a grain of sand and the largest cell in the human body.

PCOS (polycystic ovarian syndrome)   Cysts on the ovaries that may interfere with ovulation and that are characterized by low-quality eggs. Often associated with overweight patients.

PCT (postcoital or Huhner test)   Part of the initial workup when a mucus culture is taken from the woman's cervix following intercourse to determine how it interacts with sperm.

PERGONAL   An ovulation drug.

PID (pelvic inflammatory disease)   An often silent infection characterized by pelvic scarring, which is detected in about one quarter of female infertility patients.

POSTCOITAL TEST   See PCT.

PREIMPLANTATION   The first five days after fertilization.

PROLACTIN   A hormone connected to the production of FSH.

PZD (partial zona dissection)   A lab technique that encourages an embryo to "hatch" or develop prior to implantation to the endometrium.

REANASTOMOSIS   Vasectomy reversal.

REPRODUCTIVE ENDOCRINOLOGIST   Fertility doctor for a woman.

RETRIEVAL   The harvesting of eggs through the vagina in a hospital setting following fertility drug therapy in the IVF procedure.

SART REPORT   Official data from the ASRM, published bi-annually, on ART results in the U.S.

SEMEN   The male ejaculate released by the penis and consisting of sperm, fluid, and other secretions.

SPERM   Male gamete shaped like a fish with a tail and head.

SPERM WASHING   The separation of healthy sperm from seminal fluid (aka Percoll separation).

STD   Sexually transmitted disease that may lead to pelvic inflammatory disease.

SUPEROVULATION   Reaction to fertility drug therapy with Pergonal that results in the ovulation of many eggs in a single cycle.

SUZI (subzonal sperm insemination)   Micromanipulation of the sperm into the egg.

TESTICLES   Source of sperm production contained in the scrotum.

TET (tubal embryo transfer)   Embryo placement into the fallopian tube following ZIFT.

TUBAL PREGNANCY   See Ectopic pregnancy.

ULTRASOUND   A high-frequency measure of internal structures as imaged on a screen.

UNEXPLAINED INFERTILITY   The diagnosis in one out of five fertility cases.

UREAPLASMA   Microorganisms in the reproductive system that may impede sperm activity or embryo implantation.

UTERUS   The part of a woman's reproductive system that supports the fetus.

VARICOCELE   Varicosed vein in a man's testicles.

VASECTOMY   Surgical form of birth control that blocks a man's sperm ducts without interfering with ejaculation.

VAS DEFERENS   The connecting tube between the epididymis and the prostate gland.

ZIFT (zygote intrafallopian transfer)   Surgical placement of a fertilized egg(s) into the outer portion of the fallopian tube during laparoscopy before it (they) develop into embryo(s).

ZONA DRILLING   A technique whereby a hole is drilled

into the egg's shell in order to facilitate entry for the sperm.

ZONA PELLUCIDA The covering of the human egg ("eggshell").

ZYGOTE Preembryo stage of a fertilized egg.

SOURCES
(BY QUESTION)

Part I

1. American Society for Reproductive Medicine (ASRM, formerly the American Fertility Society); *Consumer Reports* (October 1996), p. 49; "Getting Started" (Resolve).
2. *Infertility: An Overview* (ASRM Patient Information Series); Dr. Lawrence Grunfeld, February 1997.
3. "Guidelines for the Provision of Infertility Services," January 1996 (ASRM); Dr. Richard Scott, ASRM 52nd Annual Meeting, press conference, John Hynes Convention Center, Boston, November 1996; Dr. Geoffrey Sher, New York, Resolve seminar, May 1996.
4. Dr. Healy, ASRM Boston press conference, November 1996; Dr. Geoffrey Sher, "In Vitro Fertilization," (*Facts on File,* 1995), p. 130.
5. Drs. Lawrence Grunfeld, Michael Drews, and Ellen Modell, "Aspects of the ARTS: A Unique Open Plenary Session," co-sponsored by the Institute for Reproductive Medicine and Science at the St. Barnabas Medical Center and the NYU Medical Center Program for IVF, NYU Medical Center, September 11, 1996; *The New York Times,* August 25, 1996, "Baby or Money Back"; "Infertility Insurance Advisor" (Resolve); ASRM FAQ #8 "State Infertility Insurance Laws" (http://www.asrm.com).

6. Drs. Alan Berkley, Ellen Modell, and Richard Scott, "Aspects of the ARTS: A Unique Open Plenary Session," NYU Medical Center, September 1996; Drs. Healy and Paulson, ASRM Boston press conference, November 1996; Dr. Donald E. Moore, "Clomiphene and Ovarian Cancer Link Studied" (*Resolve NYC Newsletter,* April 1995).

7. Dr. Sher, Resolve seminar, May 1996; Drs. Healy, Paulson, and Simpson, ASRM Boston press conference, November 1996; SART Report (*Fertility and Sterility,* November 1996); *Reproductive Times, vol. 1, issue 3,* November 1996; *Resolve Medical Updates,* Summer 1996; *The New York Times,* February 1997; Dr. Lawrence Grunfeld, February 1997.

8. See: *Unconventional Methods* (#82).

9. Drs. Berkeley and Scott, "Aspects of the ARTS," September 1996; 1996 SART Report; ASRM press release (http://www.asrm.com, November 2, 1996); Dr. Lawrence Grunfeld, February 1997.

10. Dr. Alice Domar, *Healing Mind Healthy Woman* (Henry Holt, 1996); "Mind/Body Program of Infertility" (*Fertility and Sterility, vol. 53,* pp. 246–249); "Psychological Improvement in Infertile Women" (*Fertility and Sterility, vol. 58,* pp. 144–147); Shakti Gawain, *Creative Visualization.*

11. Dr. Lawrence Grunfeld, February 1997; *The Spectator,* "The Classic Way to Have a Baby," (December 14, 1996), p. 40.

12. Dr. Alan Berkeley, "Aspects of the ARTS," September 1996.

13. Harriet Simons, *Wanting Another Child* (Lexington Books, 1995); "Better Prognosis" (*Fertility and Sterility,* p. 615, May 1986).

14. *Tubal Factor* (ASRM Patient Information Series); Dr. Neils Lauerson, *It's Your Body* (1996); *Fertility and Sterility,* January 1997; Dr. Grunfeld, February 1997.

15. *Reproductive Times,* November 1996.

16. *Myths & Facts* (Resolve).

17. *Age and Fertility* (ASRM Patient Information Series).
18. Dr. Sher, Resolve seminar, May 1996; Dr Jamie Grifo, "Aspects of the ARTS," September 1996; Dr. Grunfeld, February 1997.
19. Dr. Bert Davidson, director, San Antonio Fertility Center, "Infertility in the Large Size Woman" (*Resolve National Newsletter,* Spring 1995); "Aspects of the ARTS," September 1996; Dr. Grunfeld, February 1997.
20. Drs. Grifo and Drews, "Aspects of the ARTS," September 1996 seminar; Dr. Grunfeld, February 1997.

Part II

21. Dr. Copperman, "To Scope or Not to Scope" (*Resolve NYC Newsletter,* April 1996); Theresa Venet Grant, "Infertility Workup Includes Standard Tests" (*INCIID Fact Sheet*); *Infertility: An Overview* (ASRM).
22. *INCIID Fact Sheet,* http://www.inciid.org.; Dr. Lawrence Grunfeld, February 1997.
23. Dr. William Blank, "The Role of the Andrologist" (*Resolve NYC Newsletter,* January 1997); *INCIID Fact Sheet,* http://www.inciid.org.
24. *Male Infertility* (ASRM); Dr. Sher, Resolve seminar, May 1996.
25. *Fertility and Sterility* (May 1996); ASRM press release, April 29, 1996; *Reproductive Times,* November 1996, Dr. Larry Lipshultz, "Are Sperm Counts Really Changing?" (*Resolve National Newsletter,* Fall 1995).
26. *Male Infertility* (ASRM Patient Information Series); Dr. Grunfeld, February 1997.
27. *Husband Insemination* (ASRM Patient Information Series).
28. Dr. Sher, p. 103; Dr. Robert Winston, *Making Babies: A Personal View of IVF Treatment* (BBC Books, 1996), p. 54; Susan Treiser, *Guide to Infertility* (1994).
29. Dr. G. Sher, p. 72.
30. Dr. Richard Marrs, *Dr. Richard Marrs' Fertility Book*

(Delacorte, 1997), p. 92; Dr. Isaac Kligman, Resolve seminar, December 1996.

31. *Husband Insemination* (ASRM Patient Information Series).

32. Drs. Marc Goldstein and Zev Rosenwaks, and Linda F. Davey, "Micromanipulation Techniques Offer New Hope" (*INCIID Insights, The Newsletter of the International Council on Infertility Information Dissemination, vol. 1, issue 1,* Fall 1995); Dr. Joseph Schulman, "ICSI—A New Treatment for Severe Male Infertility" (*Resolve of the Washington Metro Area,* May/June 1994).

33. *Ovulation Detection* (ASRM Patient Information Series).

34. Diane Clapp, "What Is a 'Poor Responder'?" (*Resolve National Newsletter,* Summer, 1995); Dr. Grunfeld, February 1997.

35. Dr. Sher, Resolve seminar, May 1996; *Assisted Reproductive Technologies* (Organon patient guide); Diane Clapp, "Medical Updates" (*Resolve National Newsletter,* Winter 1996).

36. Dr. Grunfeld, February 1997; "Hysteroscopy v. Sonohysteroscopy" (Huntington Reproductive Center), ASRM poster, November 1996.

37. *Infertility: An Overview* (ASRM); Dr. Grunfeld, February 1997.

38. *Laparoscopy and Hysteroscopy* (ASRM); Dr. Grunfeld, February 1997; Dr. Sher, p. 62.

39. Dr. Lauerson, p. 343; Dr. Sher, p. 62.

40. *Ovulation Detection* (ASRM).

41. *Infertility: Coping and Decision Making* (ASRM Patient Information Series).

Part III

42. Dr. Grunfeld, February 1997; *Tubal Factor* (ASRM Patient Information Series); Dr. Sher, p. 98; Dr. Lauerson, p. 346; Dr. Marrs, p. 258.
43. Part a. "Aspects of the ARTS" seminar, September 1996. Part b. Dr. Grunfeld, February 1997.
44. *Birth Defects of the Female Reproductive System* (ASRM Patient Information Series); Dr. Lauerson, p. 318.
45. Part a. Dr. Sher, p. 90; Dr. Jamie Grifo, "Aspects of the ARTS" seminar, September 1996; Dr. Anibal Acosta, "Antisperm Antibodies" (*Resolve National Newsletter*) Spring 1996; "Phospholipid Antibodies" (*Infertility Review*, 1995, Repromedix Fertility Laboratory). Part b. Dr. Grunfeld, February 1997; Dr. Drews, "Aspects of the ARTS," September 1996; "Immune System" (*INCIID Fact Sheet*, Winter 1996).
46. Dr. Attila Toth, "The Fertility Solution" (*Atlantic Monthly*, 1991); Dr. Isaac Kligman, Resolve NYC meeting, December 1996.
47. Part a. Dr. Grunfeld, February 1997; Dr. Sher, p. 114. Part b. Dr. Kligman, December 1996.
48. Cynthia Orenberg, *DES: The Complete Story* (St. Martin's Press, 1980).
49. Drs. Grunfeld and Drews, "Aspects of the ARTS," September 1996 panel.
50. *Endometriosis* (ASRM Patient Information Series); Dr. Stephen Corson, "Endometriosis: The Enigmatic Disease" (*Essential Medical Systems*, 1992); Dr. James Liu and Dr. Marcelle Cedars, "Endometriosis: Current Concepts and Treatment" (*Resolve National Newsletter*, Winter 1997); Dr. Robert Nachtigall, "Ovarian Cysts and Infertility Treatment" (*Resolve National Newsletter*, Fall 1996); *Commonweal* study, 1996.
51. Dr. Michael Zinnaman, "The Environmental Assault on Male Fertility: Fact or Fiction" (*Resolve National Newsletter*, Fall 1995).

52. *Tubal Factor* (ASRM); Dr. Maria Bustillo, ASRM press conference, June 8, 1994.

53. Dr. Grunfeld, February 1997; *Uterine Fibroids* (ASRM Patient Information Series); *Abnormal Uterine Bleeding* (North American Menopause Society).

54. Part a. *Fertility Drugs* (ASRM). Part b. *Ovulation Drugs* (ASRM); Dr. Sher, p. 5.

55. "Preserving Your Fertility" (Resolve); Dr. Marrs, pp. 210–211.

56. P038, Huntington Reproductive Center, ASRM Meeting, November 1996; *Journal of the American Medical Association,* 12/15/96.

57. *Recurrent Miscarriage* (ASRM Patient Information Series).

58. *Ovulation Detection* (ASRM Patient Information Series); *Hirsutism and POS* (ASRM).

59. Dr. Grunfeld, February 1997; POD (ASRM); Polycystic ovaries (Organon).

60. *Abnormal Bleeding (NAMS);* Dr. Lauerson p. 355.

61. "The Nation's Most Common Infections Are Sexual" (*The New York Times,* p. 27, October 20, 1996); "Sexually Transmitted Disease and Infertility" (ASRM, press release, April 30, 1996); "Preserving Your Fertility: Risk Factors" (Resolve).

62. Menopause and Perimenopause (ASRM); NAMS Web site. http:/www.menopause.org.

63. Dr. Jessica Brown, "Early Pregnancy" (*Resolve NYC Newsletter,* January 1997).

64. *Infertility: An Overview* (ASRM).

65. Dr. Sher, pp. 9–10; *Dr. Marrs,* pp. 187–207.

Part IV

66. Dr. Attila Toth, *The Fertility Solution;* Linda Ruffin, "Antibiotic Treatment: The Easiest Cure Is Often Overlooked" (*Resolve NYC Newsletter,* September 1995).

67. Dr. Sher, p. 179.

68. Dr. Jacques Cohen, "Aspects of the ARTS" panel, September 1996, *Resolve NYC Newsletter,* December 1996.

69. ASRM poster 070, Dr. Maria Bustillo, ASRM Annual Meeting, November 1996; *Third Party Reproduction* (ASRM); Joann Paley Galst, "Are Donor Gametes Right for You?" (*Resolve NYC Newsletter,* Summer 1995).

70. Dr. Grunfeld, February 1997; *Third Party Reproduction* (ASRM).

71. Part a. *Resolve NYC Newsletter,* December 1996; Dr. Joe Leigh Simpson, ASRM press conference, June 1994 (NYC) and November 1996 (Boston); St. Barnabas prize paper, ASRM Meeting, November 1996. Part b. ASRM poster 039; Dr. Timothy Smith, "Embryo Grading" (*Resolve National Newsletter,* Summer 1995); Dr. Maria Bustillo, ASRM press conference, June 1994. *Part c. ASRM Guidelines for Practice and Ethical Considerations of ART.*

72. Part a. *Clomid—Ovulation Drugs* (ASRM); Dr. Simpson, ASRM Meeting, November 1996; Rosemary Black, "Conception at Any Cost?" (*Child,* June/July 1995). Part b. *Pergonal*—"Induction of Ovulation With Human Menopausal Gonadotropins" (*Guideline for Practice,* ASRM): Serono press release, August 1996. Part c. FSH—*Polycystic Ovaries* (Organon brochure); *Polycystic Ovarian Disease* (ASRM). Part d. *Lupron—Ovulation Drugs* (ASRM). Part e. *Progesterone—Ovulation Drugs* (ASRM); Serono press release, August 1996.

73. Diane Clapp, *Resolve NYC Newsletter,* January 1996.

74. 1996 SART Report; Dr. Paulson, ASRM Meeting, November 1996; Dr Grunfeld, February 1997; GIFT and IVF (ASRM).

75. Resolve.

76. Dr. Sher, pp. 91–92.

77. Dr. Kaylen Silverberg, "IUI Update" (*Resolve National Newsletter,* Summer 1995); *Husband Insemination* (ASRM); *Intra Uterine Insemination* (Organon).

78. Part a. Dr. Grunfeld, February 97; 1996 SART Report;

Resolve Medical Updates (*National Newsletter,* Summer 1996); Dr. G. David Adamson, "Use and Misuse of ART Statistics" (*Resolve NYC Newsletter,* September 1996). Part b. Dr. Simpson, press conference, ASRM Annual Meeting, November 1996; IVF and GIFT (ASRM); ASRM poster 039, "Embryo Quality," 1996 ASRM Annual Meeting. Part c. Dr. Paulson, press conference, ASRM Annual Meeting, November 1996; 1996 SART Report.

79. "Male Infertility: New Focus & Finds," (ASRM press release, July 15, 1996); ASRM poster 042, "Nonsurgical Sperm Aspiration," 1996 Annual Meeting; *INCIID Fact Sheet.*

80. Dr. Grunfeld, February 1997.

81. Dr. Sher, p. 153.

82. Part a. Acupuncture: Roger Hirsh, OMD, *Chinese Medicine* (e-mail: fertility@earthlink.net). Part b. Cough syrup. Part c. Imagery: Shakti Gawain, *Creative Visualization;* Dr. Andrew Weil, *Spontaneous Healing* p. 242. Part d. Dr. Grunfeld, February 97. Part e. Homeopathy: Dana Ulman, *Consumer's Guide to Homeopathy* (Tarcher, 1995); *Homeopathy Medicine for the 21st Century* (1988, North Atlantic Books).

Part V

83. Dr. Grunfeld, February 1997; Kathryn Faughey, Ph.D., "Spirituality and Infertility" (*Resolve NYC Newsletter,* May 1994).

84. "Aspects of the ARTS," September 1996; Gina Maranto, "Delayed Childbirth," (*Atlantic Monthly,* June 1995); "Pregnancy After 40" (*Town & Country,* March 1996); William Mosher and Anjani Chandra, *Family Growth Survey* (National Center for Health Statistics).

85. *Ovulation Drugs* (ASRM).

86. Dr. Kerryn Saunders, press conference, ASRM 1996

Meeting; Dr. Kerryn Saunders, et al., "Growth & Physical Outcome of Children Conceived by IVF," (*Pediatrics, vol. 97,* p. 688).

87. Dr. Grunfeld, February 1997.
88. Dr. Grunfeld, February 1997; Dr. Sher, p. 82.
89. ASRM 1995 ethics statement; Dr. Sher, pp. 135–136.
90. *Ectopic Pregnancy* (ASRM Patient Information Series); Dr. Copperman, *Resolve NYC Newsletter,* April 1996; Dr. Sher, p. 127.
91. Dr. Sher, p. 170.
92. "ASRM Statement on Unethical and Fraudulent Practices in Reproductive Medicine" (press release, July 17, 1996); *Resolve National Newsletter,* Spring 1995; *Net News,* October 1996.
93. Dr. Grunfeld, February 1997.
94. *Ovulation Drugs* (ASRM).
95. Drs. Mark Damario and Zev Rosenwaks, "Counseling and Screening for IVF" (*Resolve NYC Newsletter,* May 1995).
96. *Recurrent Miscarriage* (ASRM); Resolve materials.
97. Dr. Grunfeld, February 1997; Dr. Sher, p. 46; Dr. Jessica Brown, "Multiple Pregnancies" (*Resolve NYC Newsletter,* April 1995).
98. ASRM; 1996 SART Report; Patricia Mendell and Pamela Madsen, "Beyond Success Rates" (*Resolve NYC Newsletter,* September 1996).
99. *Donor Insemination* (ASRM).
100. Resolve National.
101. World Wide Web.

TEN KEY FERTILITY CONTACTS

1. American Society for Reproductive Medicine
   1209 Montgomery Highway
   Birmingham, AL 35216
   (205) 978-5000 or e-mail: asrm@asrm.com
   (same information for SART)

2. American Academy of Medical Acupuncture
   5820 Wilshire Boulevard
   Los Angeles, CA 90036
   (800) 521-2262

3. Endometriosis Association
   8585 North 76th Place
   Milwaukee, WI 53223
   (800) 992-3636

4. Ferre Institute, Inc. (Infertility Education)
   258 Genesee Street
   Utica, NY 13502
   (315) 724-4348 or e-mail FerreInf@aol.com

5. NAMS (North American Menopause Society)
   c/o University Hospitals, Dept. of OB/GYN
   11100 Euclid Avenue
   Cleveland, Ohio 44106
   (216) 844-8748

6. National Center for Homeopathy
   801 North Fairfax Street
   Alexandria, VA 22314
   (703) 548-7790

7. OPTS (Organization for Parents Through Surrogacy)
   7054 Quito Court
   Camarillo, CA 93012
   (805) 482-1566

8. Organon Pharmaceuticals
   800-IVF-PALS (insurance information)

9. RESOLVE
   1310 Broadway
   Somerville, MA 02144
   Helpline (617) 623-0744 or http://www.resolve.org

10. Serono Symposia, USA
    100 Longwater Circle
    Norwell, MA 02061
    (800) 637-7872

INDEX